Trager Mentastics

Trager Mentastics

movement as
a way to agelessness

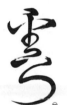

Milton Trager, M.D.

with Cathy Guadagno, Ph.D.

Foreword by Turnley Walker

Station Hill Press

Published by Station Hill Press, Inc., Barrytown, New York 12507.

Distributed by The Talman Company, 150 Fifth Avenue, New York, New York 10011.

Produced by the Institute for Publishing Arts, Inc., Barrytown, New York 12507, a not-for-profit, tax-exempt organization.

Design plan by the authors, Milton Trager and Cathy Guadagno, with realization by Susan Quasha and George Quasha. Production assistance by Richard Gummere and Bryan McHugh. Staff support by Christine Miller, Frauke Regan, and Paul Woodbine.

Cover design by Susan Quasha.

Cover photograph by Daniel L. Fishman. Acknowledgements for other photographs appear on page 174.

The words Trager ® and Mentastics ℠ and the Dancing Cloud calligraphic logo are service marks of The Trager Institute and are used here by permission. These marks, either individually or together, may only be used to describe the professional services of members in good standing of The Trager Institute.

AUTHOR'S ACKNOWLEDGEMENT

The author wishes to thank and acknowledge the Trager Institute—the Instructors, Practitioners and Students. [M.T.]

Library of Congress Cataloging in Publication Data

Trager, Milton.
  Trager mentastics.

  1. Exercise. 2. Mind and body. I. Guadagno, Cathy.
II. Title.
RA781.T73 1987   613.7'1   87-23454
ISBN 0-88268-048-X

Manufactured in the United States of America.

Contents

This book is dedicated to the two women in my life
who made it all possible.

Foreword

The man comes first and then his work. It was noted long ago, and often since, that a great writer is simply a great man writing, who has made writing his chosen work and the carrier of what he has to say and, more important, what he is.

So it is with every man who has done distinguished, valuable and, in the deepest sense, helpful work.

So it is with Milton Trager, M.D., who is much more than *Medical Doctor,* an honorable designation to which he has brought unusual and perhaps unique honor.

The boy, the man and the life were highly unusual and perhaps unique long before the key accomplishments began. A poor boy from the toughness of Chicago's streets and less advantaged neighborhoods, driven from schooling far too early by work-for-a-living necessities, having at first only his own *body* to elevate his life, becoming a dancer and then a professional boxer.

In each of these endeavors, he began and continued to learn, by intuition and by some special magic that was always in his mind and *hands*, how to *tune* the body, how to hook it up with mind and spirit, how to repair it when damaged.

A particular greatness was developing in young Milton Trager long before the harrowing academic and intellectual struggles required to develop and release his genius-touched abilities. Those struggles to regain lost education, and to continue all the way through medical school and further professional training, came when other men were relaxing into middle age. They were epic struggles—and triumphs.

Following this, the key work of his life continued to grow outward from the greatness that was always there. His tuning of minds and bodies, his *hooking up* the whole of the individual into a more soundly functioning, joyful, creative, fuller person, has become his life work—his art—and more recently his teaching.

Fame, which he has never sought, has followed him, and reached him, and this, too, will grow.

His new book, *Trager Mentastics: Movement as a Way to Agelessness,* represents a key part of his teaching. Its profound value is that its values can reach and help everyone who reads it. It is practical *and* inspiring. It can be the reader's hook-up with a man whose greatness began and developed through his lifetime, and now continues to culminate in his work.

Turnley Walker

Mr. Walker is the author of seven books, including *Rise Up and Walk* and *The Presence of Mine Enemies.*

First Steps to Mentastics

Body Waves

All movements on the earth—waters, winds or living creatures—follow the undulating curvature of a wave. Sound and light exist as waves with specific frequency and length. Mentastic movements create wave-like shimmerings that resonate through the body and have a loosening and lightening effect on both the body and mind.

An ageless body is one that gracefully moves through space. It remains true to its wave-nature with movements that are flowing and confident, not rigid and cautious. The body is carried along comfortably, its posture naturally aligned without appearing bent and defeated under stress and the pull of gravity. Such a body is beautiful at any age!

Mentastics is an approach designed to restore and maintain this agelessness of body and mind. The term is a coined expression meaning "mental gymnastics"— very gentle gymnastics that are mentally directed to free the body from tensions.

One of the most pleasing and natural aspects of Mentastics is the way the body's own weights are used to open and move each part. For example, the arm can hang and swing freely, joining—not resisting—the effects of gravity. Movements done in this manner can bring us into a deeply relaxed and peaceful state that Dr. Trager calls "hook-up."

Hook-up is the same as meditation. Dr. Trager describes its process as blending and becoming one with the energy force that surrounds all living things. Science has been able to observe and even measure this energy. We can see and study it through the use of scientific instruments, such as Kirlian photography, illustrated later in this book. Most important, we can *experience* hook-up. When in hook-up, we can enjoy a renewed and enhanced sense of well-being.

Getting Started

Mentastic movements are done with ease and simplicity. Let's experience the quiet, yet dynamic, feeling of Mentastics:

Stand or sit in a comfortable position and just let your arms hang freely at your sides. Now slowly and without tension raise one hand in front of you as though you are about to strum a guitar. Gently play the guitar and feel the weight of your thumb as it bounces freely. You will feel the weight of the thumb about halfway up to the wrist. Now ask yourself, "What can be lighter? What can be softer?" Let these questions direct the movement and notice how they affect the feeling in your hand. Allow your hand to become even lighter. Notice how your movement becomes refined as it responds to the message from your mind.

Now continue this same strumming movement, and let your arm hang down from your shoulder, keeping it close to your leg or chair. Feel the weight of your thumb and the shimmering of the tissues in your arm. Do not *try* to make the tissues shimmer. It will happen if you do not make an effort. If you feel stiffness or rigidity in the movement, slow down and resume asking, "What can be lighter? What can be freer?" And ask these questions in a way that does not demand an answer—only suggests a sensation.

Now pause a moment. Feel the difference between your two hands, arms and shoulders. Notice what impact a little bit of softness can have on the body/mind. The tingling sensations and gentle pulsations are signs of your own aliveness! The deeper you feel and play with the weights of your body, the quieter your mind will become.

This is just a beginning. Yet even this simple movement can be done again and again, first with one arm and then with the other arm, with profound results. It is meditation-in-motion and can be done anytime, anywhere.

Hook-up is the basis and primary goal of Mentastics. It is a natural state of being. Sometimes when walking in the woods or by the ocean we become very quiet and feel "connected" with our environment: it's that simple. We become one with the rustling leaves or the waves dancing in and out—*allowing* us to come into a feeling of peace.

Getting Results

Mentastics have stood the test of time only due to the consistent results that so many people have experienced. Dr. Trager first discovered Mentastics over sixty years ago as a teenager working out on the beach. Once a thin, frail child, he gradually became fascinated with the way the body functions and the satisfaction and pleasure he felt when moving in an effortless rhythm. He soon saw the positive changes Mentastics could make in the quality of people's lives. This encouraged Dr. Trager to continue to devote his time to develop his approach. He was profoundly committed to his work and confident of its future, yet he could hardly have foreseen its great impact.

It was not until 1975, at California's famed Esalen Institute in Big Sur, that Dr. Trager's innovative approach to bodywork and movement first surfaced into full public view. The demonstration he gave at Esalen deeply stirred his audience and aroused the interest and commitment necessary to expose his work to a larger audience. Workshops, and, shortly afterwards, an institute were formed to preserve and extend his teachings. This led to the full-scale training program that has grown so impressively over the last decade. Today there are over 1,000 certified Practitioners and professionally-oriented students throughout the world.

I became one of those students, and it was in 1979 during an intermediate level training that I had the good fortune to meet Dr. Trager. What I had heard about him had an almost legendary quality—tales of wisdom and wit, his healing hands, his creativity, genius and dedication to serving others in need. What impressed me personally was his direct and sensitive manner, embodied in his famous Trager "touch"—a light, yet penetrating, hands-on contact. His presence was at once powerful and peaceful. This rare combination of attributes comprises the unique quality of the work he teaches—the Trager Approach, consisting of gentle manipulation by an experienced Practitioner on a bodywork table, and Mentastics, the movements done by an individual either separately or as an adjunct to the tablework.

I came to this book out of my experience of *getting results* from Mentastics. I love doing them every day, and they allow me to keep my body free of aches and pains. They have altered my posture and enhanced the grace, ease and coordination of my walking, dancing and swimming. It is reassuring and pleasurable to experience increased well-being even as I grow older. This daily renewal is what Dr. Trager refers to as agelessness.

Mentastics is a daily practice that can benefit virtually everyone. These movements can aid recovery from a wide range of specific ailments. In my private therapy practice I have seen Mentastics bring inspiring results in cases of physical pain and trauma, including lower back syndrome, stroke and whiplash, to name a few. It has been wonderful to see results even with difficult conditions such as Parkinsonism. By incorporating Mentastics into their daily lives, they lose much of their rigidity and improve their balance.

The book has been written in a "verse form" intended to simulate how Dr. Trager's teachings are presented in his workshops. The first part, "Essentials," gives Dr. Trager's account of the development and basic principles embodied in Mentastics. The second part, "Mentastic Movements," is a practical introduction to actually doing them. We urge you to read the book in its present order so you may approach Mentastics with a sense of awareness and enjoyment.

For further instruction in Mentastics, a video tape will soon be released. Information on classes in Mentastics that are being taught internationally can be obtained by writing or calling the Trager Institute (see the last page of the book).

How much lighter and freer can you be? Put yourself in motion as you embark on a playful discovery. In the simplicity of Mentastics lies its beauty as well as its challenge.

I will always carry with me a feeling of profound gratitude for Dr. Trager and his work, which has enriched and expanded the horizons in my life. Mentastics is a dynamic and effortless avenue towards creating a more loving and peaceful world for ourselves and our children.

Cathy Guadagno, Ph.D.

Preliminaries

The only purpose and value
of all of the words in this book are to
stimulate your desire to
explore through movement
a unique approach to self-development and
psycho-physical integration.

Trager Mentastics is for those
who are seeking something
    better and deeper for their
body and mind.
Mentastics can open a new door into the
realm of feeling.
Feeling is the core and essence of
Trager Mentastic movements.

Each of us can develop and
more fully realize who we are
only when we experience something
different and better.
Who we are is the sum total of
every feeling experience,
    mental and physical,
    positive and negative,
that we have ever had in our lives.
These feeling experiences are stored in the
    unconscious mind and
    cannot be erased.

Whenever I use the word "feeling,"
I am referring to the unconscious mind.
   The conscious mind does not feel.
The unconscious mind is the part of our mind
that is not conscious.

Mentastics is a coined expression meaning
   "mental gymnastics."
They are mentally directed movements that
suggest to the mind feelings of
lightness, freedom, openness,
grace and pleasure resulting in
   an ageless body.

   Mentastics can reverse the ageing process.
It begins very early in life, usually around age 10.
As we age, it is not the tissues of the body
that are at fault.
The rigidity that one feels as one gets older
is from the effects of the many adverse experiences
that have occurred during one's life.
These experiences can include trauma,
illnesses and disappointments.

The tensions, restrictions and rigidities
responsible for the ageing process
   are not physical patterns,
   but are mental patterns.

Generally, more stiffness is found in older people
because they have had more time to
accumulate faulty patterns that are more
deeply instilled in the mind.
For these people, and for those with severe trauma,
it will take more time and more patience to
    discover and find
    the freedom of their body and mind.

Agelessness is not the same as youthfulness.
Youthfulness is for kids.
An ageless body is a free and open and comfortable body.
Mentastics offers a short-cut to this freedom.
By experiencing more joy through movement,
one can experience more joy in life.

These movements are very simple.
And yet many of my students view their simplicity
    as a challenge.
That challenge is a personal exploration toward their own
    self-development.
To develop means to constantly search and find
that which is better for the body and mind.
    Development is a never-ending process.

You will be able to learn Mentastics from this book if you
    DO NOT TRY. TO TRY IS TO FAIL.
There is no effort or design. There is no technique.

Every moment of every movement is a chance to
develop the mind as well as the body.
Once you begin to develop a habit of searching for
that which is freer and better by asking,
    "What is lighter? What is freer than that?,"
you will be doing Mentastics.
It is a subtle process that brings one into a
peaceful, meditative state that I call
    "hook-up."
Hook-up brings refined sensitivity and
meaning to the movements.

It is not possible to do Mentastics perfectly.
It is the approach towards perfection
that is meaningful.
The greatest rewards and benefits in doing
Trager Mentastics are
freedom and agelessness.

I
ESSENTIALS

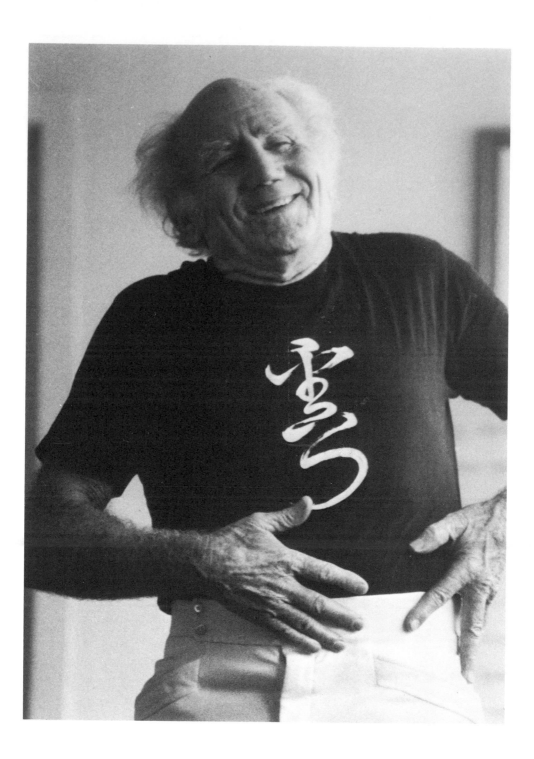

The Birth and Development of Trager Mentastics

Mentastics was a quiet discovery in my life.
   It was a happening.
The subtle feelings of these simple movements
are so pleasurable that
I have continued to move and develop this approach
for over sixty years.
The awakening process, which allowed me to be
aware of my body,
was initiated with
   the taking of ONE DEEP BREATH.

In 1924 my family moved from Chicago to Miami, Florida.
To help the family, I took a job as a mailman.
I was only 16 years old at the time, with a rather frail body.

In the post office there was a large bulletin board.
We were required to sign our initials to indicate that
we had read messages about taking care of our feet or
taking care of our eyes, etc.
Then one day there was a sign on the bulletin board
about taking care of the chest that said,
    "Take a deep breath."
I read the sign and initialed the paper.

The next day there was no one around and
I saw the sign again.
   "Take a deep breath."
So I put down my mail sack, paused a moment,
and took a deep breath.
   That was the beginning of me.
I felt myself intimately for the first time.
   And that felt great.

This first deep breath has meant much to me,
      and has helped me in
      helping others.
In Chapter 10, you will experience
      how the breath is utilized
      to create an expansiveness in the chest.

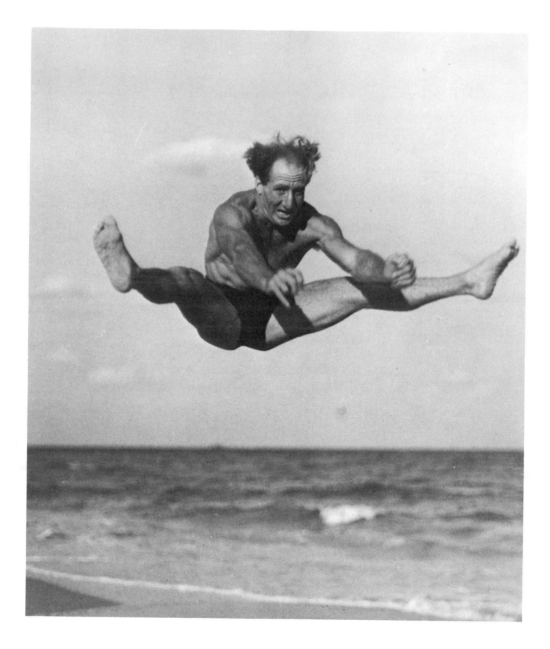

In 1925 I was transferred to the beach area
where I could run and learn gymnastics.
Having a muscular body was important to me.
I became an acrobatic dancer,
loving to do leaps and aerials, and
    the feeling of motion inside of myself.
Everyday after work I would go to the beach to train.
It was always just before sunset,
    with the beach deserted.
The only sound one could hear was
the water coming in and
    splashing upon the shore.

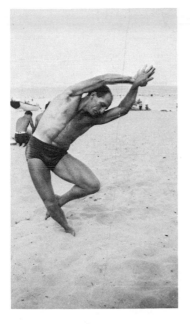

I would fall into a rhythm with the ocean as
I would swing my arms.
This sense of Oneness with the waves
would bring me into a
finer and finer state with a feeling of
        perfect peace.

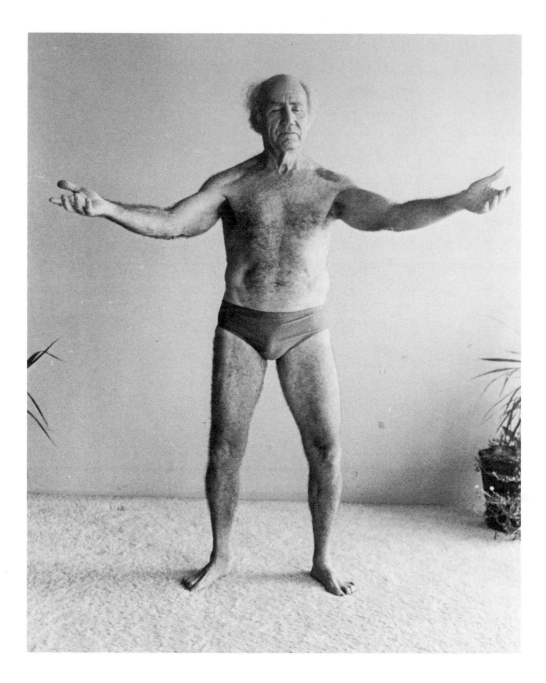

I call this natural and harmonious state of being.
    "hook-up"
because, as in meditation,
one connects with the energy force that
surrounds all living things.
    Hook-up
is the most basic
and important ingredient
    in Mentastics.

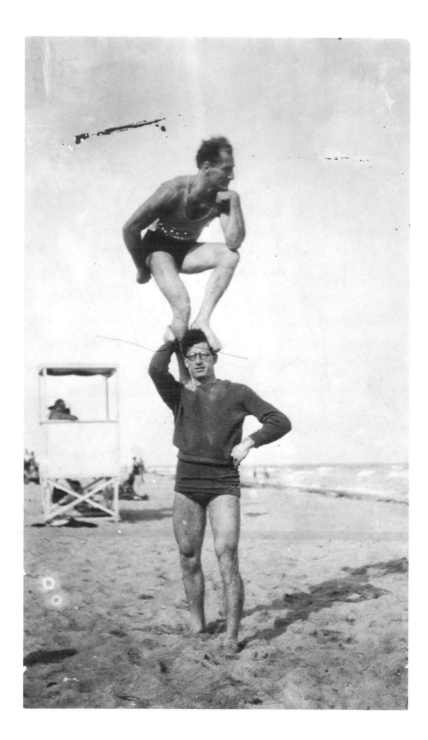

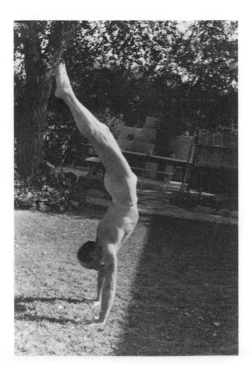

This movement and meditation became
a daily part of my life.
I continued doing acrobatics every Sunday
    with my brother, Sam,
on the hard sand after the tide would go out.
One day Sam said,
    "Let's see who can jump the highest."
Then, from nowhere, I said,
    "Let's see who can land the softest.
    What can be softer?"
This simple question opened up my mind to
new possibilities of how to perform other movements in
    an effortless manner.

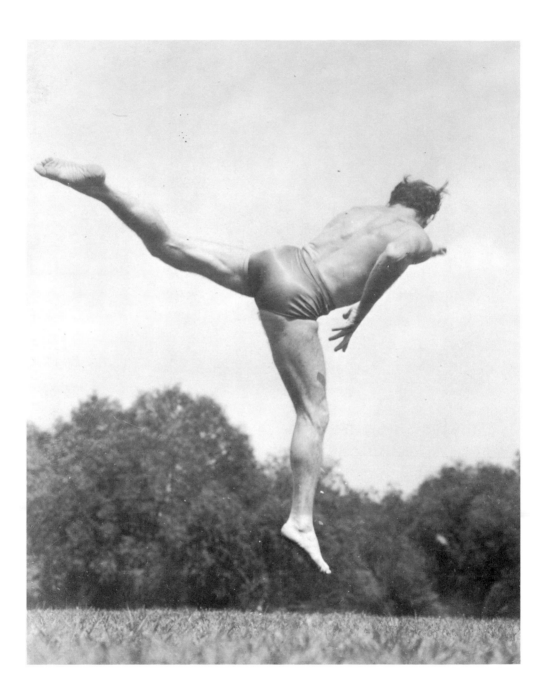

To jump high takes force. One must build up a
        physical feeling and
give it all one has to perform the movement.
        This is effort.
To land softly means that one must ask,
utilizing one's mind to direct the movement,
questions such as,
        "What is softer... and
        what can be softer than that?
        What is lighter... and lighter... and
        lighter than that?"
This process is the basis of Mentastics.

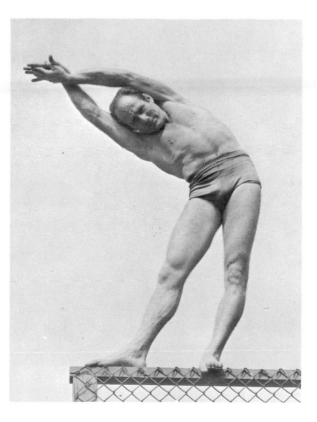

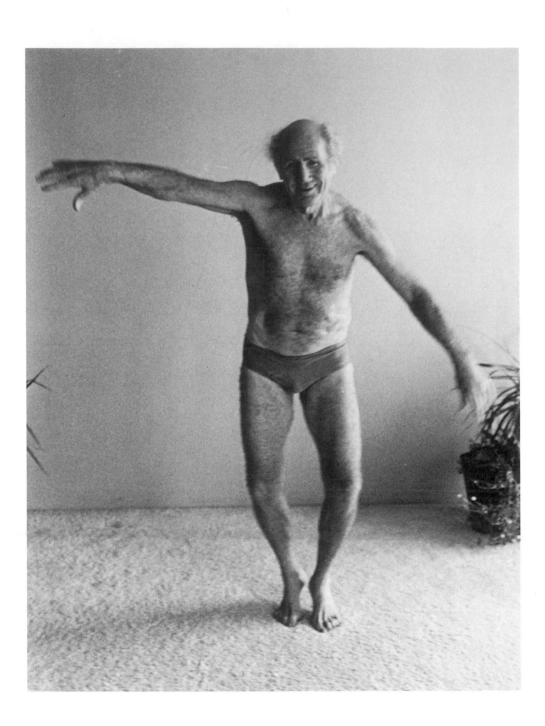

For over five years I wore and
carried my muscles around
with exaggerated tension
until my body responded to the
    freer and finer feelings that
my mind picked up from doing Mentastics.
I developed a Mentastics warm-up routine that
I would teach to a group of male acrobats at the beach.
We would begin with the
    arm and leg Mentastic movements
as described in later chapters, and
create other movements that
my body felt like it needed at that moment.

Even today, I do Mentastics in this manner.

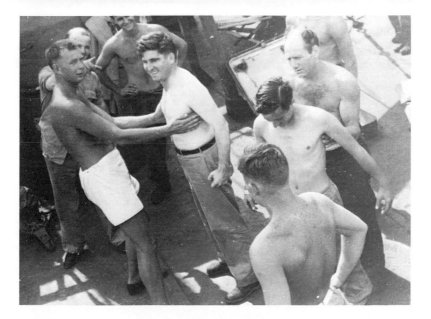

Dr. Trager (top right) teaching Mentastics during World War II aboard a landing ship, L.S.T. 314, Bizerte, North Africa.

As you walk, jump or do any movement
in a manner that is softer,
    you must bend the knees.
The knees absorb the shock so that the entire body can give.
The development of my professional boxing and
professional dancing was based on this principle.
There are no jolts, jarring or sudden movements.
The movements originate from the mind,
    not the body.

And it all starts by asking questions such as,
    "What is lighter?
        What is softer?
            What is freer?"

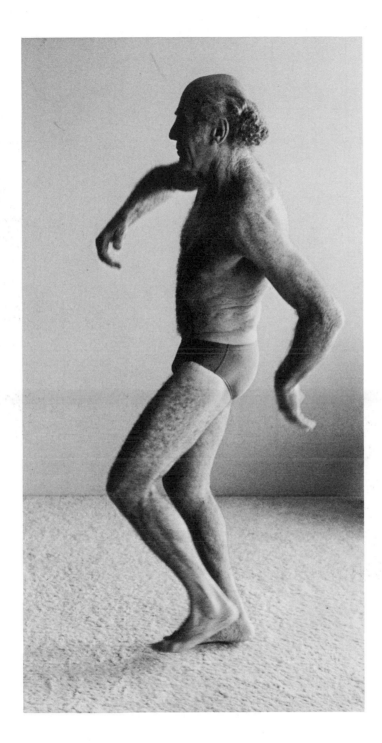

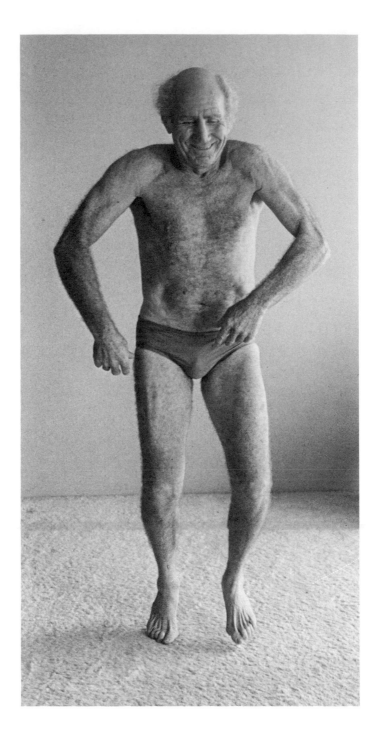

These movements were not called Mentastics
until a long time later.
Then, in 1974, my wife, Emily, and I
coined the term
    "Mentastics."
She thought of "mental" and I came up with "gymnastics."

I have been doing Mentastics for
over sixty years because
the movements pleasure me.
I know that if you allow Mentastics to become
a part of the way you live,
that you will derive much satisfaction and enjoyment
    from your body and mind
    for the rest of your life.

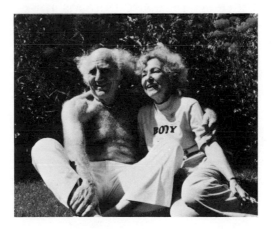

The Principles and Philosophy of Mentastics

Mentastics is an indirect approach for
releasing blocks and tensions.
One must bypass the conscious mind and
allow the movements to be
    directed from the
    unconscious mind.
My students and patients often ask,
    "What is the unconscious mind?"
My reply is always the same.
The unconscious mind is the
    part of our mind
    that is not conscious.

Every feeling experience you have ever had
is stored in the unconscious mind and
    cannot be erased.
Since there are no erase buttons in
the unconscious mind,
all of its information regarding
    feelings, perceptions,
    memories and understandings
is at our disposal to be tapped and utilized
like the data stored in a computer.
It is our most powerful resource.

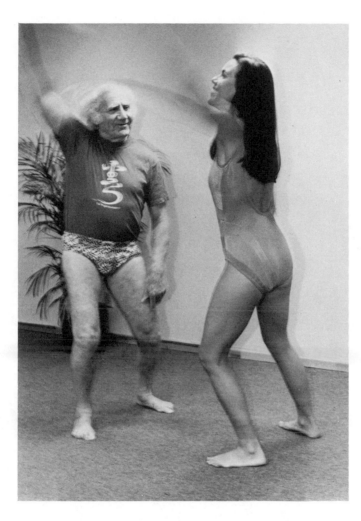

This also means that one does not have to
    "get rid of" anything
in order to develop into a more fully realized person.
One can simply add more
positive experiences to one's life.
This can happen by doing Mentastics.

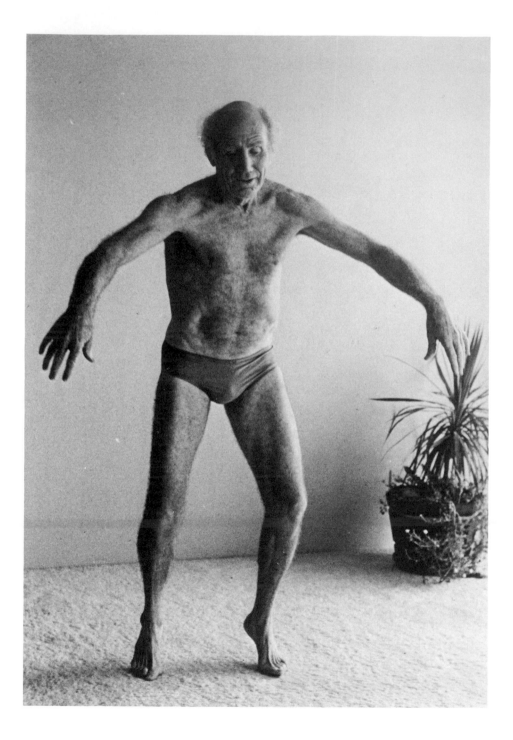

Mentastics do not consist of a
technique, method, or a routine.
It is an APPROACH of
    mind and motion
    perfectly synchronized.

Mentastics are never about how many,
    how fast, how far or
    how physically powerful the movements are.
Mentastics are done with the feeling of
    how light, how beautiful, how free,
    how complete the movements can be.

What keeps the body restricted is not
a true physical block,
    but a mental pattern block.
It is the MIND that unconsciously directs
the function of the body.
    THE BLOCKS EXIST IN THE MIND.

The body is quite dumb.
An example of this is that
    Fred Astaire's feet are dumb.
It is what he has developed in his mind that
allows his feet to move
    so effortlessly.
When Mentastic movements are
directed from the mind,
they become a form of
    self-expression.

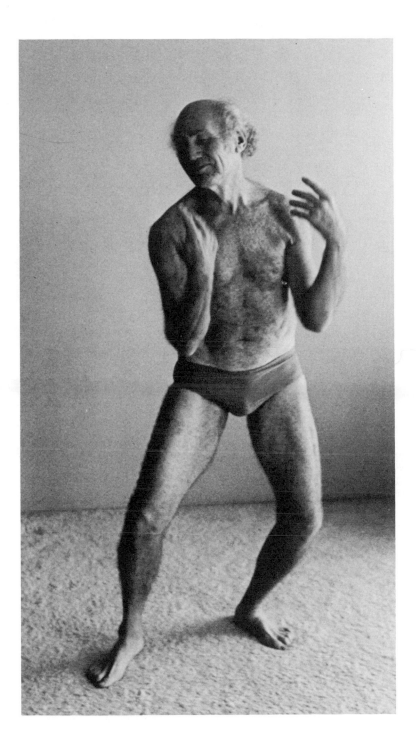

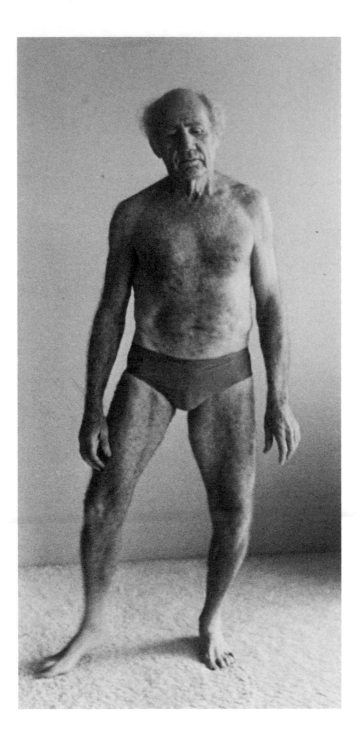

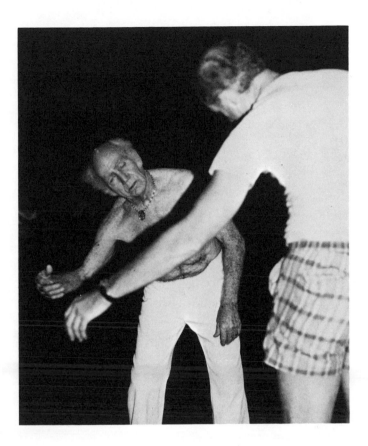

There are two basic principles in doing Mentastics.
The first and most important principle is what I call
   "HOOK-UP."
When one "hooks-up" with
the energy force that surrounds us all,
then one comes into
   a finer state of being.
It is a feeling deeper than relaxation.
   The feeling is Peace.
Hook-up creates a flow and a rhythm.
   Hook-up is like meditation.

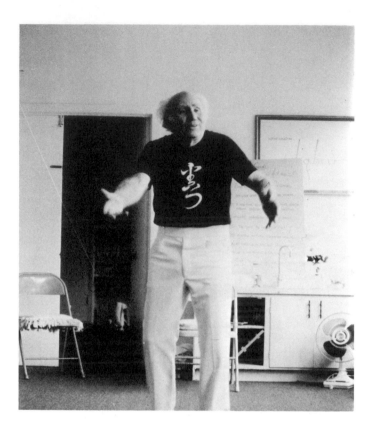

The second basic principle of
Mentastics is to
    ALLOW THE MOVEMENTS TO HAPPEN.
    DO NOT TRY.
To try is an effort, and effort creates tension.
Play with the feelings of how loose,
    how free, how nothing.
    Be patient.
Do not try to accomplish anything.
    Consciously stay out of it.
    Become a part of the feeling.

When you feel tightness and stiffness
in your body
do not attack it and
do not try to make it freer,
which is the natural reaction for
the majority of people.
THE TIGHTER THE INVOLVEMENT,
THE LIGHTER THE MOVEMENT MUST BE.

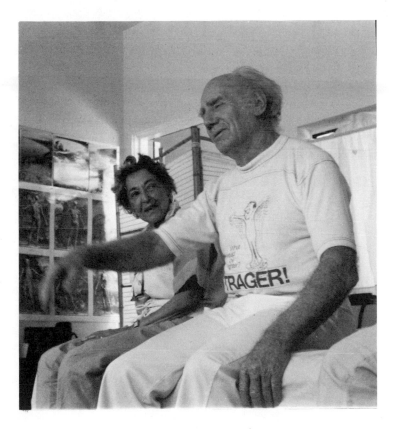

It is important that the movements be
     directed from the mind.
The process begins by
asking questions such as,
     "What is lighter? What is freer?
     What is softer?
     What is more beautiful?
     What is better?"

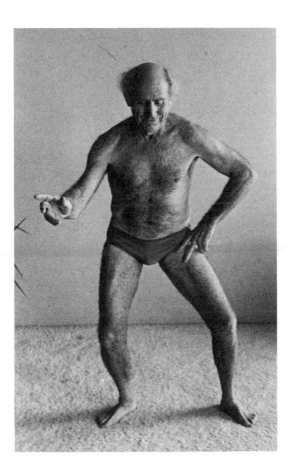

Ask the questions in a soft,
undemanding manner in which you
expect the answer to come.
By asking, you are developing the
power and potential of your
unconscious mind.
This process takes no more effort than a thought.

If you feel pain, discomfort or fatigue
while doing Mentastics, then
allow the movement to become lighter,
decrease the range or amount of movement,
slow down the tempo of the movement or
stop the movement and rest.

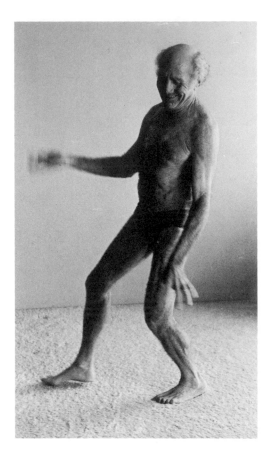

When you do Mentastics, you can experience
a more beautiful way of
feeling, knowing and
moving your body.
These feelings of freedom
accumulate and establish a
positive picture pattern
in your unconscious mind
of how much freer and softer you can be.

All of these feeling experiences
can be recalled at any time
    simply
by using the same process you use when asking,
    "Well…how does that song go?" or
    "What is my telephone number?"
This is all information you automatically retrieve
    from the unconscious.
    Recall strengthens this position of freedom
    in the unconscious mind.

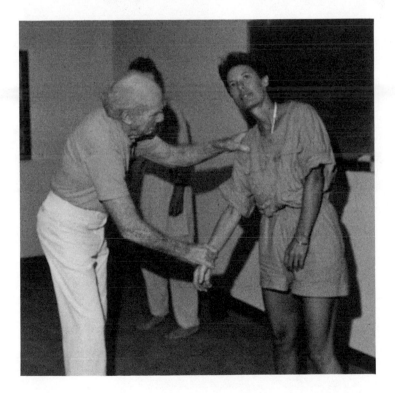

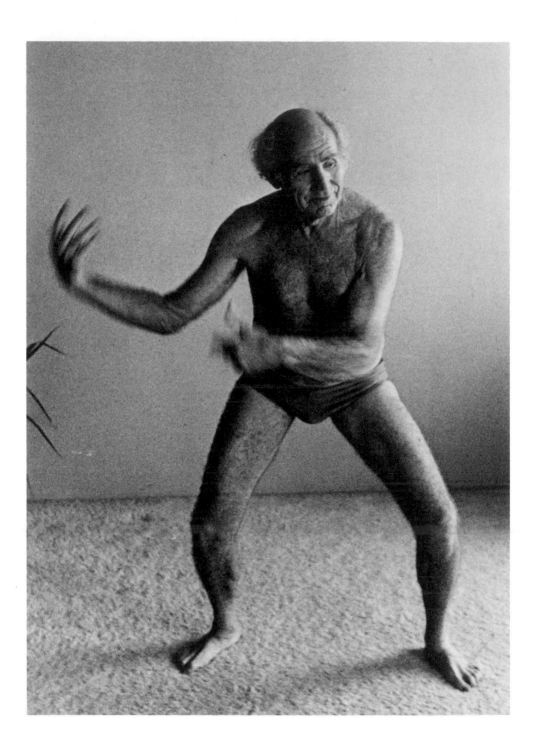

Do not analyze the movement.
Analyzation is a process of the conscious mind.
Feel the weight of whatever part of the body
you are moving.
If you are having trouble feeling the weight,
you might ask,
    "What is heavy?
    How heavy can my arm feel?"
Or you can slow the movement down.
Moving too fast will also
    bring one out of
    hook-up.

Mentastics can help develop patience.
Play with the resistance offered.
If you feel tightness,
then the needed feeling is lightness.
    What is lighter?
Take time to feel the subtleness sink in.
You will always be rewarded for your patience.

As you are doing the movements, you may think,
  "It can't be this easy.
  I am barely doing anything physically.
  And yet, I feel a change has occurred."
It is a personal, intimate experience.
It is a happening of the moment.

There are no deliberate movements.
There is no wasted motion.
  Every little movement,
  every bounce of the muscles,
  every thought
approaches a feeling of freedom and
creates an intimate integration between
the body and the mind.

The philosophy manifesting in Mentastics is a way of life.
The softness and ease that
you develop through Mentastics
can be transferred to
other areas in your life.
Through this educational process,
the movements will become automatic.
   Live the movements.

There is no limit in the development of the mind as
there is no limit to the feeling of the body.
Self-development is
   a never-ending process.

I tell my students all the time that
you can only give to others what
you have honestly developed
   within yourself.

Mentastics can never become boring because
they bring about a
    pleasurable feeling in
    the body/mind.
It is an art; and like any other art,
    practice can bring about
    beauty and form.

One cannot try to achieve excellence.
    To try is to fail.
    By being in hook-up,
the movements will flow and
become a natural part of oneself to where
    the instrument and
    the person become One.

The instrument in Mentastics is the body,
and the mind is the conductor.

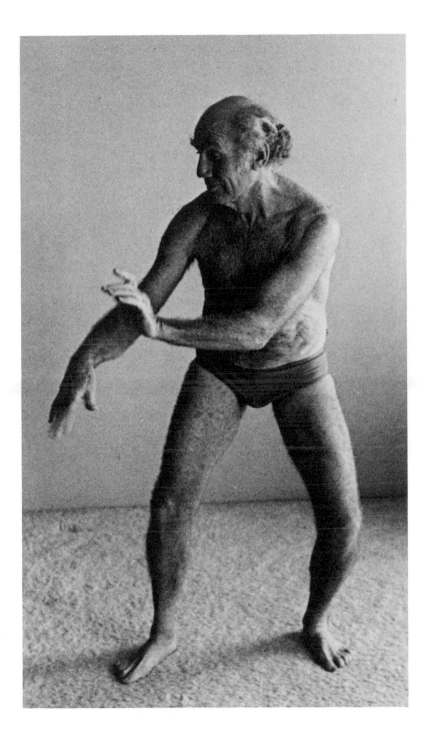

Hook-up —A Meditative Process

We are surrounded by a force;
    a life-giving, life-regulating force.
It might be electro-chemical; electro-magnetic.
    Whatever. We know that this force exists.

We don't have to go a fraction of an inch
away from our body to get it.
You are enveloped by this force.
    ALLOW this force to enter.
There is no trying. There is no effort.
    To try is to fail.

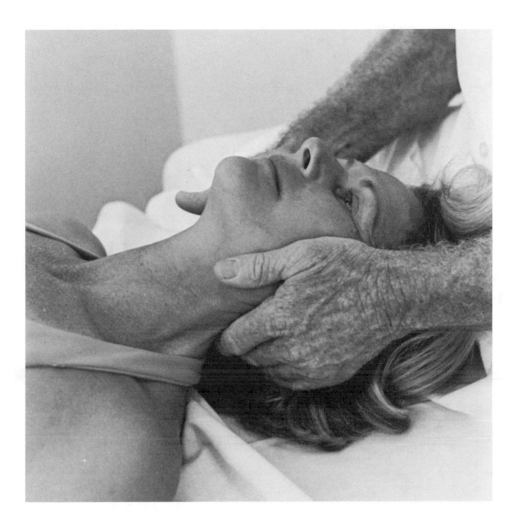

Hook-up is the same as meditation.
And like meditation, there are many levels.
One can go deeper and deeper into
a state that is beyond relaxation.
A step beyond relaxation is Peace.

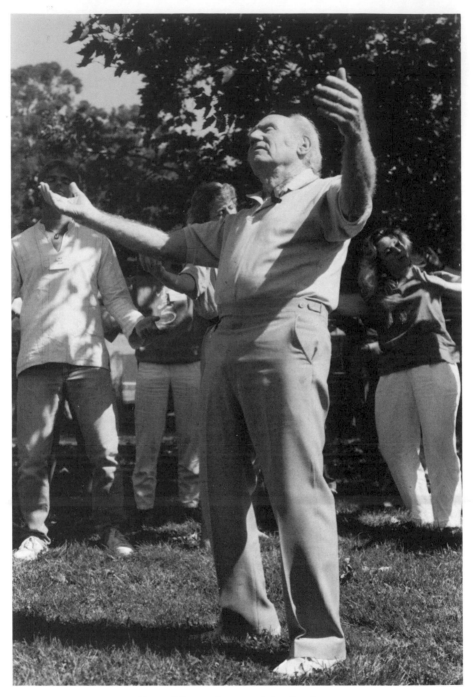

Group Mentastics sustaining hook-up.

Hook-up is not a passive state.
It is dynamic, alive, vibrant; yet peaceful.
There isn't anything one has to do to hook-up
except to allow it to happen.
Even learning and trying to let go is an effort.
    There is no effort.
    There is no design.

Just spend more time walking about
with the knowledge that
you are enveloped by this force.
You are surrounded by all of this help.
The only reason why more people are not
helped by this force is
because they are so full of
tension, worries and anxieties.

You have already experienced hook-up
at one time or another,
or many times.
You see a rainbow, a landscape, a seascape,
or a new-born baby's face.
You are struck by the beauty,
leaving you practically speechless.
If you were to talk, you might say,
    "No artist could ever paint what I am seeing."
At that moment you are in hook-up.

Or you can look out the window at a cloud.
The shape or how it is moving is not important.
If you don't see a cloud, pick out a flower
or any other object of nature.
Be part of it; until you and nature become One.

Hook-up is like basking
in a vast ocean of pleasantness.

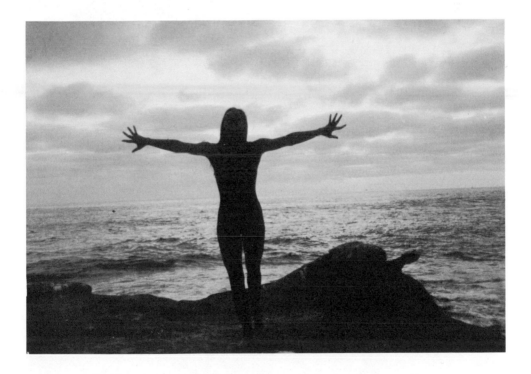

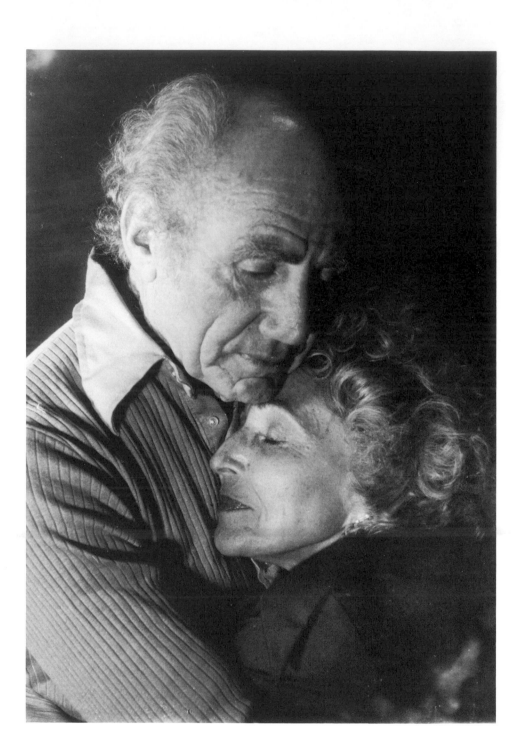

Hook-up is a natural state of being.
Do not make it special or mystical.
 For me, it is like meditation.
 For others, it is similar to religion.
It is Peace. It is a perfect state of being.

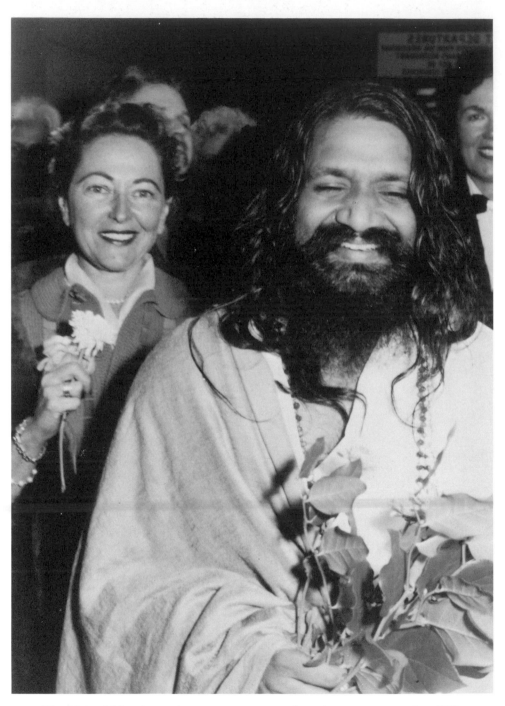

The Maharishi and Mrs. Emily Trager, his confidential secretary, spring, 1959.

In 1958, I was initiated by the
    Maharishi Mahesh Yogi,
    (who introduced
    Transcendental Meditation to the Western world)
as one of the first eight initiates in the United States.
I talked to him about Mentastics and
hook-up to which he said,
    "It is natural to go to the
    state of greater happiness.
    Whenever you are in hook-up,
    you are in the superconscious."

When you really experience hook-up,
your projection of peace to
everyone around you will be such that
they will be influenced and
respond to your vibrations.
There are few things greater than
the feeling of response.

People will want to be around you,
or help you out more simply because
your projection of joy and ease will be contagious.
    Hook-up is like the measles;
        you catch it from someone who has it.

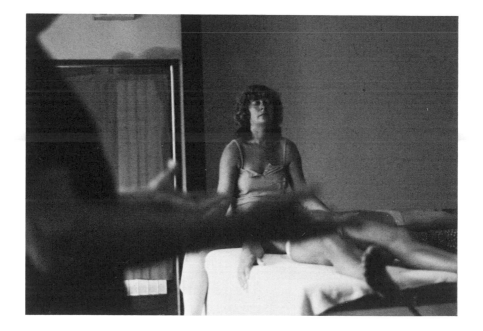

Our projection is how people judge us.
When one walks down the street,
   snap judgements are
unconsciously being made about
the people passing us.
Instantly, just by looking at a person, we may think,
   "What a lovely person" or "I'll stay away from him."
The only thing that is happening is that
we are responding to their vibrations.

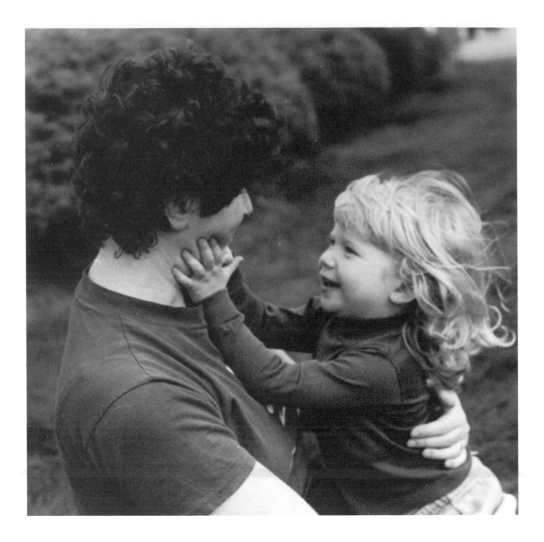

Children raised in a family where
there is hook-up can
experience and express more open
    love and communication.
If we can instill
    positive feeling experiences
in our children, then their attitudes,
outlook on life and
    self-esteem will be positive.
Their positive vibrations will attract the
    positive vibrations of others.

Hook-up can be a tool for them to use so that
they may effectively
cope with the stresses that
exist in our environment.
It is a small, yet significant step towards
    peace in this world.

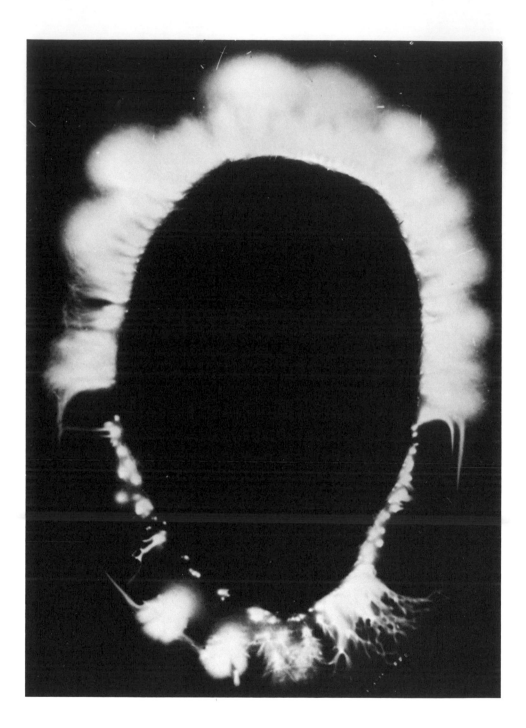

In 1975 I was invited by Dr. Thelma Moss
to come to U.C.L.A. to
participate in a study of healers
using Kirlian Photography.
Kirlian is an electrophotographic procedure
developed in 1939
to measure energy fields of living matter.

One very important thing that
I must add in relating this story is that
I do not consider myself to be a healer.

This first picture was taken of my thumb
before I started working.
The light area denotes my energy field.
I was told to work on a woman,
using my approach of
Psycho-Physical Integration,
as described in Chapter 7.

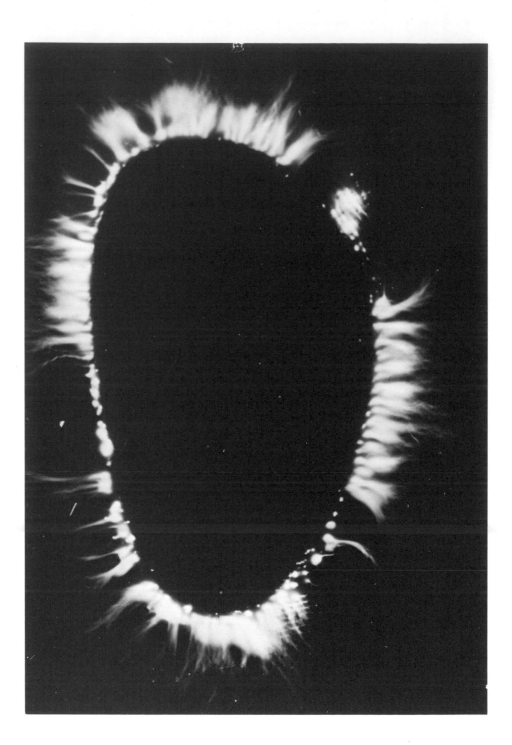

The room was dark and full of people.
I had to use a psychiatrist's couch
in lieu of a table,
which was very uncomfortable as
I had to sit on the hump of the couch.
Fatigue was setting in, and I knew that
I was not doing a good job.

After twenty minutes of working
in this draining situation,
the second photo was taken.
The picture indicates a depletion of my energy.

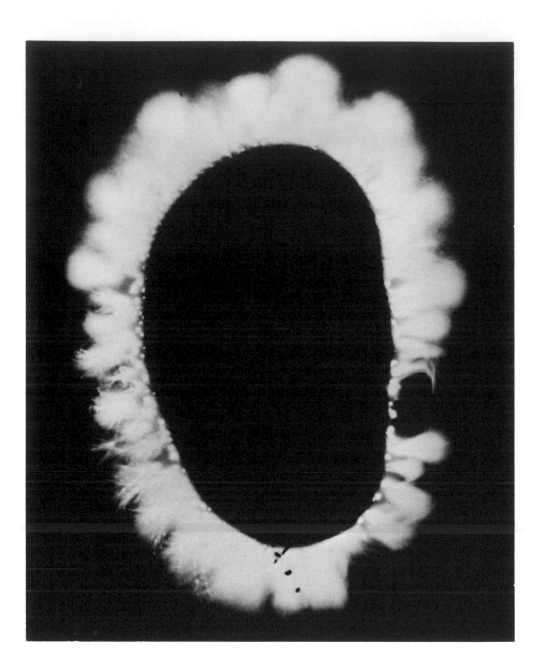

At that time I had no idea of what
the first two pictures looked like,
as they were all given to me
at the end of the day.
But following the taking of
the second picture, something inside of me
asked for a third picture to be taken;
which I did request.

Before shooting the picture,
I went into hook-up
for about 45 seconds,
and then raised my hand to indicate I was ready.

This third picture illustrates
    an increase in my energy field;
    better than when I started.
This vibrant energy force registered in the picture
    surrounding my thumb
    is hook-up.

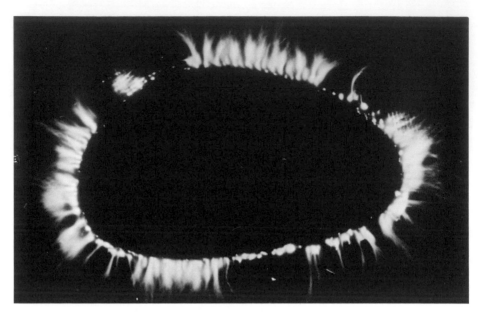

Before hook-up.

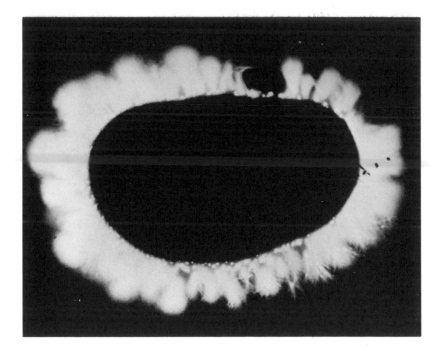

Hook-up.

76

The first step for going into hook-up is
to acknowledge that
there is a force greater than yourself.

It can be measured. We know it exists.

The second step for going into hook-up is
to allow it to happen.
Do not try to make it happen.
To try is to fail.
Trying is an effort, and effort creates tension.

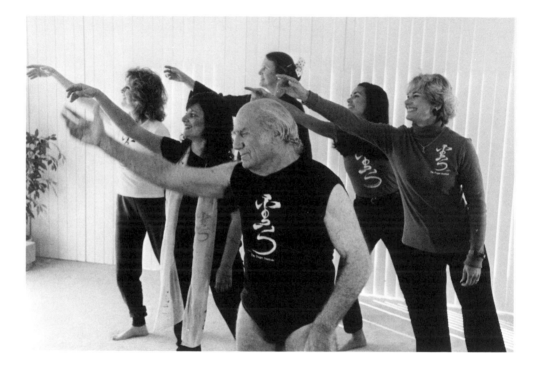

Hook-up is the most essential element of Mentastics.
Through hook-up, Mentastics can reach a point of
meditative motion as the movements become
     effortless and rhythmic with
     a dance-like quality.
One can sense and feel a new and desired
     lightness and agelessness that
     pleasures the body.
One can become intimately aware of
one's body as the mind becomes
     a subtle participant in
     every movement.

Your degree of development in
     Mentastics
depends on your depth of development in
     Hook-up.

Relaxation —A Feeling Experience

It is common knowledge among medical doctors that
one of the primary causes of
disease and illness is stress.
Heart disease, ulcers,
migraine headaches, and lower back syndromes
are just a few of the problems
directly related to unresolved stress.

Stress is unavoidable in our society
as it exists today.
However, there are some very simple and
available approaches that
you can practice in order to cope
with the stresses that surround us all.

Trager Mentastics is one such tool.

TENSION ORIGINATES IN THE MIND.
The body reflects the
degree of tension that
exists in the mind.

Maintaining excess tension consumes a lot of energy
that could be used for
other normal bodily functions.
Respiration, circulation and sleeping patterns
are all diminished and
affected by surplus stress.

A rigid body has restricted movement.
This also restricts one's ability to fully live and
enjoy life.
Movement is basic to awareness.
Doing Mentastics and being in hook-up
regulates all systems of the body.

What is relaxation?
Relaxation can never be anything but a
    feeling experience.
Just as tension is produced from inside of ourselves,
relaxation can also be produced in the same manner.
And it all starts with
experiencing hook-up so that one may
    change and develop.

Every moment of
every mentastic movement
can serve this purpose.

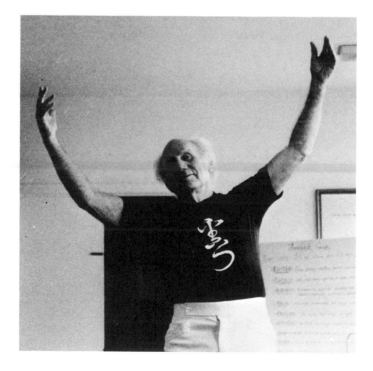

Our negative feeling experiences
  cannot be erased.
When doing Mentastics,
every shimmer of the tissue is sending a message to the
unconscious mind in the form of a
  positive feeling experience.
It is the accumulation of these positive patterns that can
offset the negative patterns
  to where the positive can take over.

When the tension and blocks are released,
  one experiences
    more energy and a greater sense of
      aliveness.

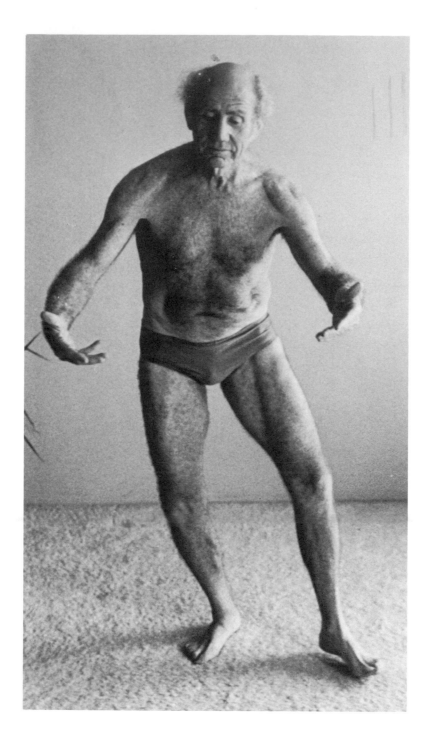

Hook-up is the key to relaxation.
Just the feeling of the weight of your arm
   can bring you into a
deeper and better
   state of hook-up.
The ultimate power of hook-up is that
this feeling of peace
can be recalled in an instant and
   at any given moment.

We can only *approach* the ideal state for our
body and our mind.
   Perfection does not exist.
It is the process that is important in
learning the feeling of relaxation.

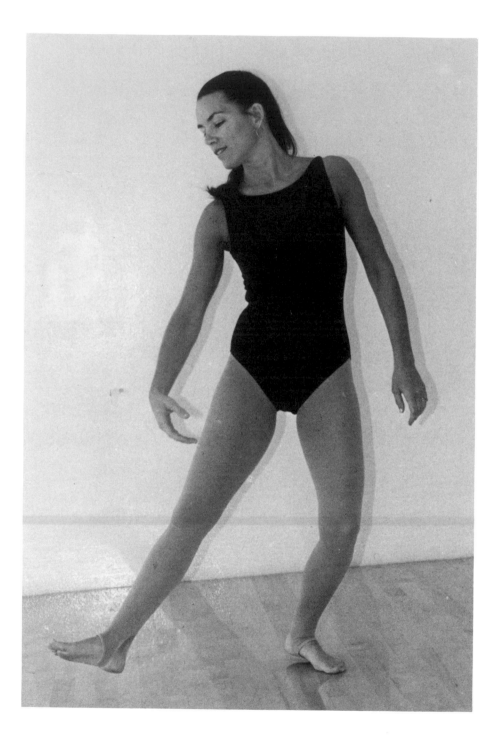

When doing Mentastics,
let the movements come from your mind by asking,
   "What can be lighter?… and lighter than that?
   What can be softer?… and softer than that?"
When you feel that the movement is softer,
then you are just beginning.
   Recall these feelings. Do not demand.

During your day, or at work, or
in any situation where you feel tense,
simply recall the feeling of lightness that
you experienced in doing Mentastics, and
you will come into a state of relaxation
to the depth in which you have developed
the feeling of relaxation in your mind.

Be patient.
It takes no more effort than a thought.
And this feeling of relaxation can be yours
   whenever you need it
   for the rest of your life.

The Application of Mentastics to Sports and Injuries

One of the most natural ways to reduce tension
is through physical activity and sports.
But the joy and expressive quality of
these activities are often
    diminished due to effort.
Lack of awareness or ignoring
    warning signals from the body
        can result in
            pain, injuries and frustration.
Most people discontinue exercise programs
    due to boredom or injuries.

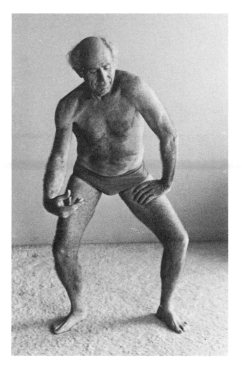

MENTASTICS ARE NOT EXERCISES
THEY ARE MENTALLY DIRECTED MOVEMENTS

The goals for Mentastics and exercise
   are not the same.
In exercise, one pursues
   increased tone, strength,
   endurance or speed.
This takes effort.
The goal of Mentastics is hook-up.
Personal feelings of
   freedom, lightness or softness
are developed within oneself.
This is an effortless process.

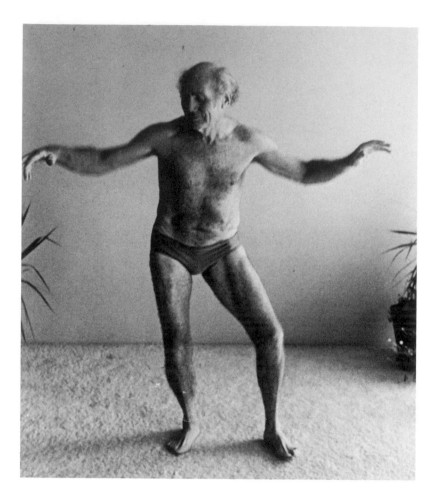

Mentastic movements are not based on the
principle of contraction
but rather on expansiveness.
One can sense and feel a new and
desired lightness that
pleasures the body.

When the muscles are over-used in
exercise or sports, a by-product called
    lactic acid is produced.
This muscle soreness is usually accompanied by
muscle fatigue that can cause the body to
    COMPENSATE.
Compensation means that other muscles must
take over doing an activity,
which increases the possibility for
injuries to occur.

Even when a person is walking
with a pebble in their shoe,
compensations occur all the way from
    feet to head.
Whenever you have an injury or excess tension,
the entire body must
    compensate and accomodate.

The soreness and achiness acquired from
too much activity
    usually lasts 24 to 48 hours.
Continued soreness or acute pain is
    an indication of injury.

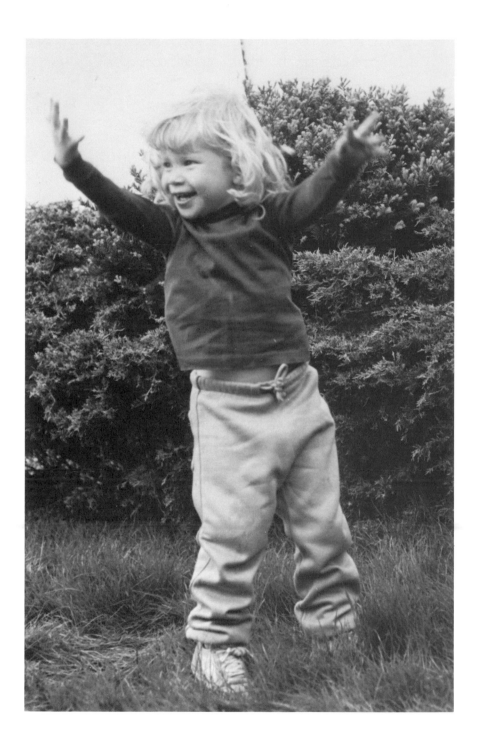

So many people are only aware of their bodies
when they feel pain.
The body itself does not experience pain.
    Pain is registered in the mind.
The route of pain goes from the injured area,
through a multitude of stations in the nervous system,
    to the mind.

Mentastics can be very effective in
eliminating pain in the body/mind.
Play with the tension or pain you feel.
Do not try to get rid of it.
The tighter or more painful the area is,
the softer you must become.
If any of the movements in this book
seem too difficult,
you can adapt and modify the movement
until you find success.
    Play and discover.
    Find your own way.

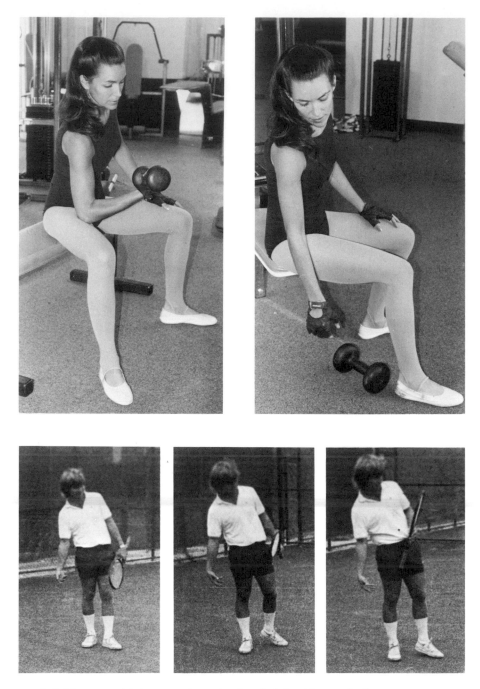

Bob Blaze, world class tennis professional, doing Mentastics between serves.

Mentastics can balance and counteract the
strenuous effects of
   weight lifting,
   jogging and
   other physical activities.
One can create a simple, light feeling
within oneself, so that
less energy expenditure is required in the activity.

Here are some examples:
before and after each serve,
   a tennis player can do arm Mentastics;
before diving in the water,
   a swimmer can do arm and leg Mentastics;
before and after curling a free weight,
   one can do arm Mentastics;
before hitting a baseball,
   the player can open the chest, back and arms;
before dancing,
   one can do Mentastics for the entire body.

Mentastics can also be a tool for
transforming rigid, clumsy movements into
flowing and pleasurable movements.
The feelings of grace and openness can be
developed through Mentastics,
You can derive much pleasure from
movements that are graceful.

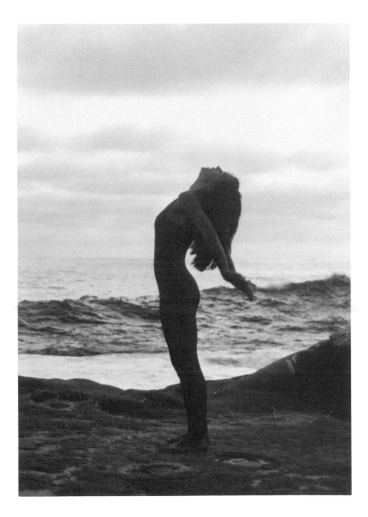

Being in a state of Hook-up
allows the practioner to "work" on a body
    with sensitivity and
    without fatigue.

Mentastics can aid in developing a
responsiveness and integration
    between the mind and body,
preparing and warming up the body for
    more vigorous activity,
relaxing the mind,
preventing injuries,
maintaining the position and condition of a
    flexible body/mind, and
promoting self-awareness.

The development of lightness is in the mind.
    The development of coordination is in the mind.
This development is limitless.

Mentastics as an Adjunct to Psychophysical Integration

Soon after the evolution of Mentastics,
an event occurred which transformed my life.
That event led to the discovery and development
of the companion work to Mentastics that I named
    Psychophysical Integration,
      or simply the Trager Approach.

It is a hands-on approach in which
    my mind transmits a message of
    lightness or freedom to my hands,
which are working on the tissues of my patient.
The practitioner knows when the patient's mind
has received the message
    by the response in
    the patient's tissues.
It involves the transmission of feeling messages from
    my unconscious mind
      to their unconscious mind.

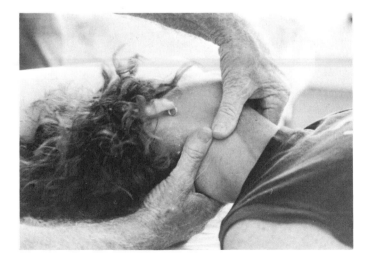

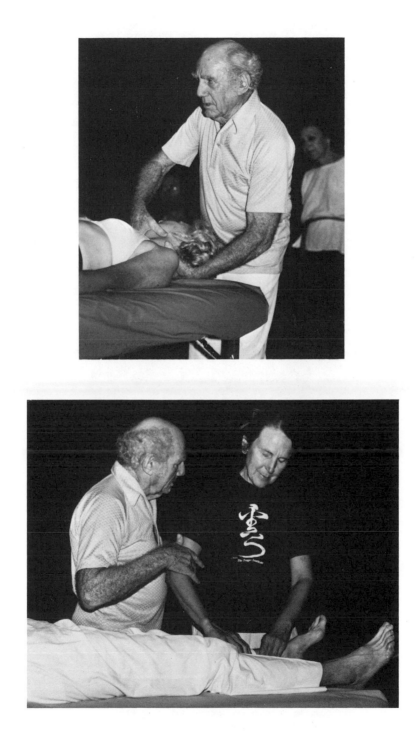

I was almost 18 and in training to become
a professional boxer.
Everyday after working out, my trainer,
Mickey Martin,
would give me a massage to relax my muscles.
But one day he looked very tired,
so I told him to lie on the table.
I had never touched anyone in this manner before,
but my hands started to do movements that
seemed helpful and relaxing to his body.

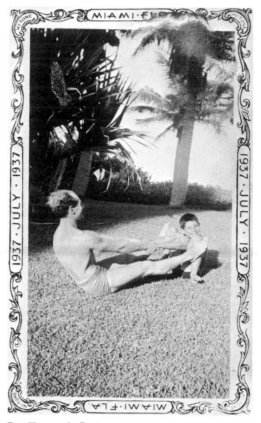

Dr. Trager's first experience working with a spastic, whom he succeeded in getting to walk (Miami Beach, 1937).

100

Mickey turned over after a few minutes and said,
    "Hey, kid. Where did you learn how to do this?"
    I had no idea what he meant as I replied,
    "From you, Mickey."
He said, "I've never done anything like that to you.
    I'm telling you,
    you've got hands."

After Mickey finally convinced me that
    I "had hands,"
I went home and worked on my father,
who had been suffering from
sciatica for two years.
After the session, his pain went away and
never came back.

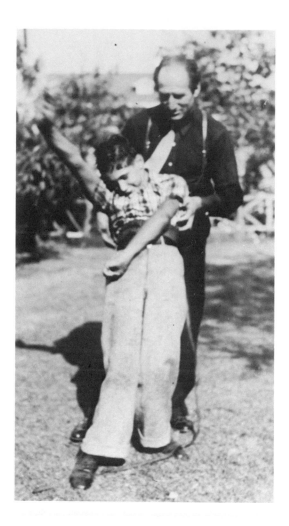

I developed a curiosity to find out if
what I was doing could also help others.
My first clientele consisted of
polio and paralysis cases.
I would work on the children at
the beach or in the neighborhood.
This was during the time of the polio epidemic.

When I was 19, my first polio client walked
after having been paralyzed for four years.
The results were so encouraging that
    I continued to develop
    Psychophysical Integration.

In 1977 I closed my medical practice in
Waikiki, Hawaii
to devote the rest of my life to
demonstrating and teaching
practitioners and instructors
Psychophysical Integration and Mentastics.

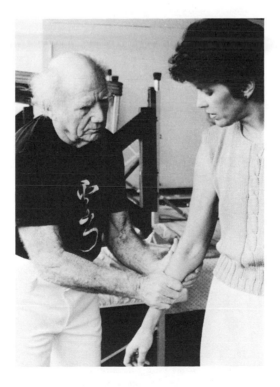

Mentastics is an adjunct to
    Psychophysical Integration.
I tell my patients that the
Mentastic movements I teach them are
    AS IMPORTANT
as the tablework session.
It is a tool that they can use
whenever they feel the need
without having to depend upon the therapist.
Mentastics can maintain the body in an
    open position and
    pain-free condition.
It is like doing the Trager tablework on yourself.

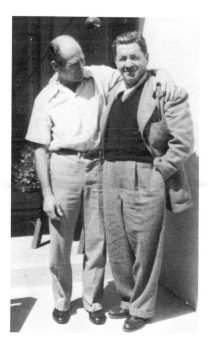

**Dr. Trager and "Curly" of the Three
Stooges, following a session in
Psychophysical Integration (circa 1947).**

The goals and principles of
Mentastics and Psychophysical Integration
are the same.
The basis is hook-up.
The feelings are lightness and freedom
    without pain.

The tablework movements of the practitioner are
directed by hook-up.
The practitioner feels the response in
the patient's body.
At that point the patient becomes the therapist.
The practitioner is only an instigator.

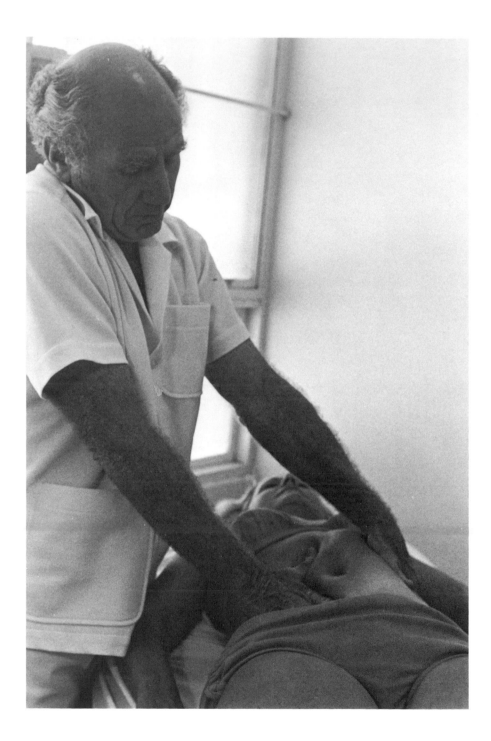

People often ask,
    "Dr. Trager, why do you do this work?"
The answer is simple.
I do this work because of the
    TISSUE RESPONSE that
I feel in others.
The response is such a
rewarding and satisfying feeling.
I feel the change in the body and
sense the change in the individual.

Hook-up is the key ingredient in promoting change.
Everytime you hook-up, you grow and
develop a little bit.
Development takes place in the unconscious mind.
My work promotes the development of a person as a
    mental/physical being, or
    Psychophysical Integration.

Problem Backs

In my private practice doing
Psychophysical Integration,
I have worked on
thousands of cases of problem backs,
and 90 per cent have only needed
one tablework session.
The reason for this success is that Mentastics have
maintained their backs in an
    open position and
    pain-free condition.
This is how powerful these simple movements can be.

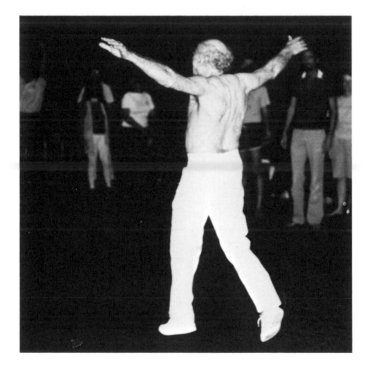

I have a congenital back problem called
    spondylolisthesis.
In my case the body of the fifth lumbar vertebra
has slipped forward over the sacrum which caused
strain on the muscles in my lower back.

So many of the Mentasics movements were developed
out of my need for an approach to
keep my back pain-free.
I can do practically anything with my back.
I am aware that the problem is there, so
    I do Mentastics every day.

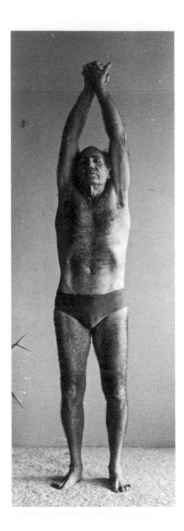

Mentastics have helped me so much
and are such an integral part of my life,
that I do them automatically whenever I am
    walking,
        getting up out of a chair,
        or reaching for a glass off the shelf.

I will never need a back operation
due only to the freedom
I am able to maintain in my lower back
    by doing Mentastics.
I am one of the few medical doctors who
do not prescribe strengthening exercises
    for problem backs.

Once you have had a chronic problem
with your back,
you will always have a
    "problem back."
However, this condition
does not have to limit your activities.

Mentastics can be your best friend for life.
    Do them everyday,
    and anytime during the day
    whenever you feel the need.

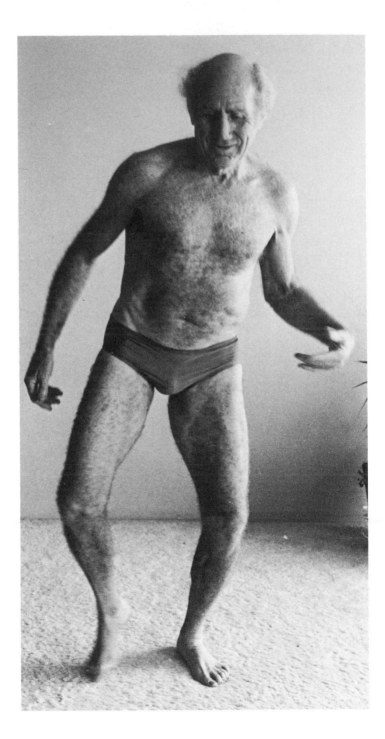

Mentastics can be incorporated into your daily life.
If you have been lifting heavy items,
     gently do the arm Mentastics
to relieve the tension and fatigue.
If you have been sitting in a chair
or driving a car for too long a time,
get up and
     gently do the kicking Mentastics
to relieve the stffness.

Sitting in an automobile will
generally aggravate a lower back problem.
For those who spend a lot of time driving,
I advise placing
a wedge-shaped automobile seat cushion,
sitting on the thick portion of the cushion,
or a rolled-up towel
     in the space
     between the seat and
     the back cushion.

Do not try to get rid of the pain or stiffness
by "driving it out."
When Mentastics are done in hook-up,
new and positive feeling experiences will
overpower the old, destructive patterns.

Play with the movements.
Feel the pleasure in the
simple bouncing of your muscles.
Mentastics is a way of
    celebrating the aliveness
    that exists and
    can be developed in the body/mind.

II
MENTASTIC
MOVEMENTS

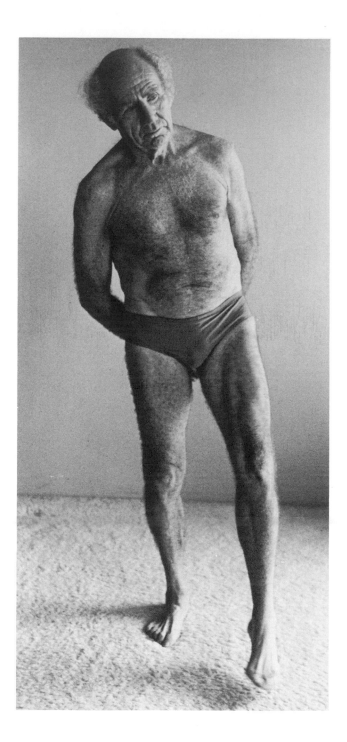

Kicking the Legs

One of the most important Mentastic movements
for the lower back is
kicking the legs.
It is also helpful if you suffer with
pain or discomfort in your knees.
I teach this simple kick to
every patient that I see,
even if they do not have a problem with their back,
because it will prevent a problem from setting in.

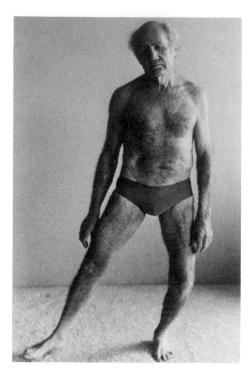

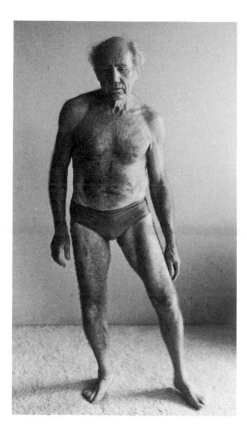

Kick each leg once to each side in a manner
so that you can see and feel
your thigh muscles bounce.

Keep the foot close to the floor,
or just barely touching the floor.
This will prevent contraction in the hip
and allow you to feel
the weight of your leg.

Kick with the subtle feeling that your leg is
falling down and out of the hip socket.
Feel the shaking in your calves and ankles.

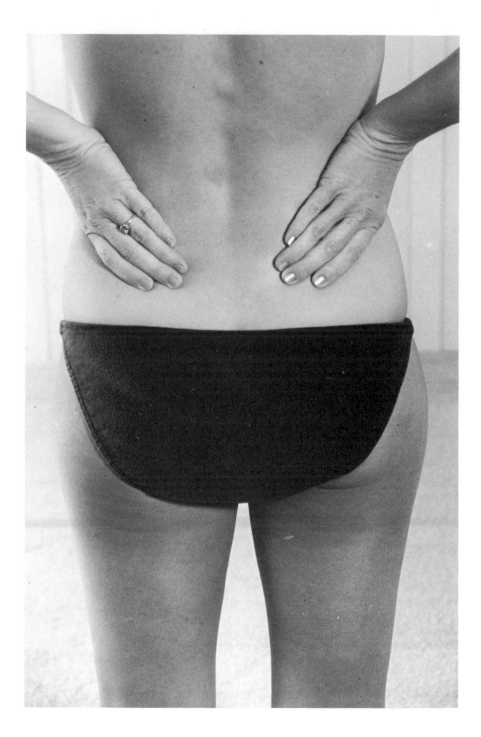

This movement creates an
easy, natural,
little jiggle
in the lower back
which can radiate up past the middle back,
which can also relieve general tension.

You can feel this jiggle by
pressing your fingers on the
bony structure of the lower back.
The bounce you feel in the lower back indicates a
release of the articulation
in the lumbar area.
Without the bounce, the kick is meaningless.
Do not try to make it bounce.

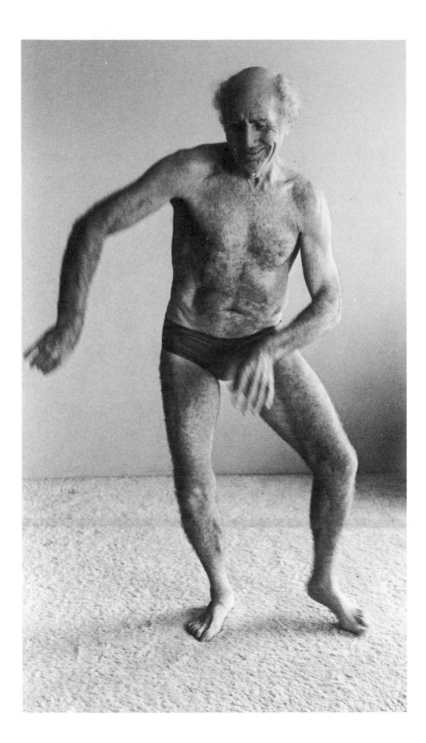

Continue to kick while walking as if you are
kicking a tin can.
It is done with an attitude of indifference,
as though you do not care
where the can goes.
Take small steps without sustaining the kick.
If you feel tension developing in your thighs,
then you are holding the foot out too long.
With every step you take in this manner,
you can be creating
    space and freedom
    in the lower back.

It is never how strong you can kick.
Do not drive the legs out.
    The kick is not a deliberate movement.
    It is like doing nothing. It is a happening.
    Feel the jiggle in your lower back and legs.
    Let it be rhythmic, beautiful, and expressive,
    like a dance.

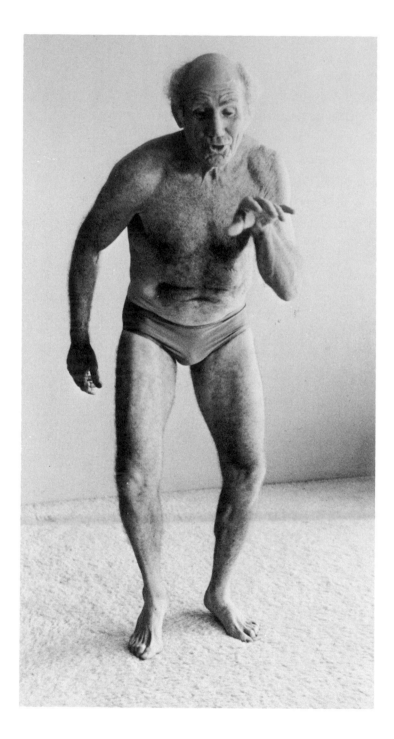

As you continue walking and kicking,
be aware of how you feel.
If you feel tired,
    then stop the movement and rest.
If you feel pain,
    then that is a signal that
    you are using too much effort.
Slow down and
allow the movement to
originate from your mind by asking,
    "What is free?
    What is light?
    And lighter than that is...?"

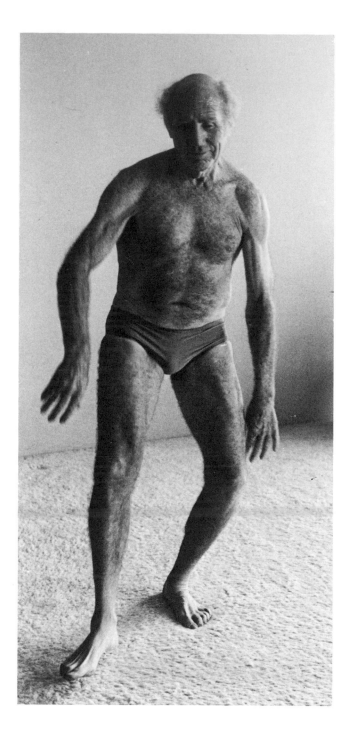

126

During your day,
as you walk from one room to another,
repeat the kicks
    with a finer feeling.
With every kick,
you will develop more and more feeling of
softness which will deepen your
    feeling of hook-up.
For many people with chronic pain
in their lower back,
the Mentastic kick is the only tool they need to
    be free from pain.

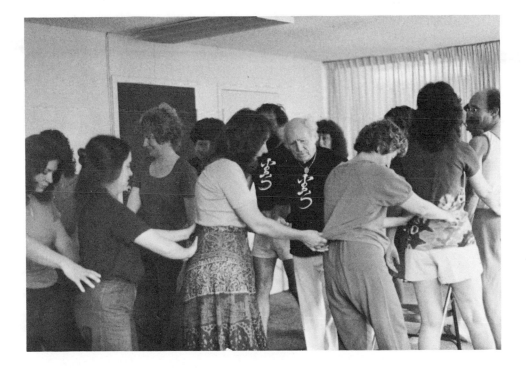

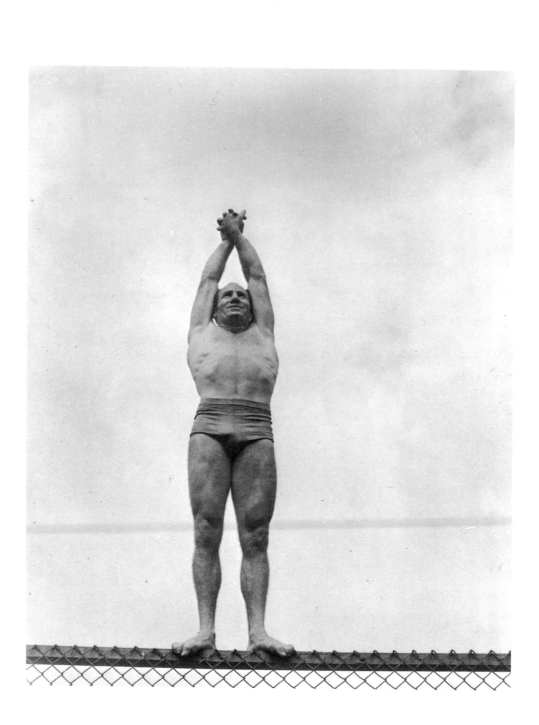

Elongation Without Strength —Proper Posture

Our posture reflects our attitudes
regarding ourselves and life.
Poor posture is not only unappealing,
but it can result in
straining muscles due to compensation.
The back muscles become tense
due to their increased work load,
and the chest assumes a closed, contracted state.

A common command while growing up is,
    "Stand up straight."
Many people associate erect posture with
    sticking the chest out,
    pulling the shoulders back,
    and sucking the belly in.
This unnatural position of the body
can only be maintained with a
    strained, continuous effort.

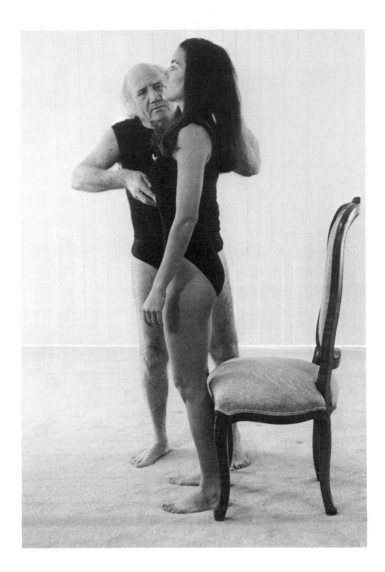

One simple way to develop elongation
is to practice
getting up and down out of a chair while
utilizing your breathing.

Begin by placing the equivalent of
a hard kitchen chair for firmness
in a space where you also have room to walk.
Stand in front of the chair so that
the backs of your legs
touch the edge of the chair.
The height of the seat should be
above the level of the knees.

Start to exhale,
and as the air continues to go out, sit down.
By allowing the air to carry you down,
the movement becomes
smooth and graceful.
To rise out of the chair,
    lean forward slightly,
    inhale and stand up
    as if the air is taking you up.
You are now in your own
    PERSONAL, PERFECT POSTURE

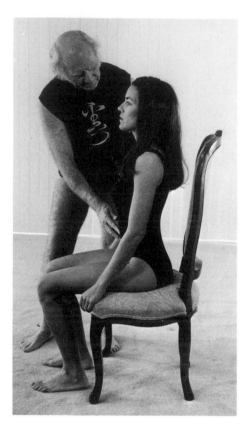

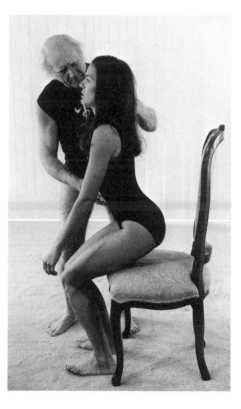

Repeat this sequence in a rhythmic manner
several times.

Exhale as you sit down.
Your air comes out in rhythm to the descent.
Feel your thighs taking you down.
There is no strain on the back.

Inhale as you rise out of the chair
into an elongated position.
Do not hold yourself in this state of elongation.
Just be up there mentally and comfortably.
Let your legs dangle from the hips,
as if you are a puppet.

Become part of this feeling of elongation.
    Enjoy!
Tension will dissolve as you come into hook-up.

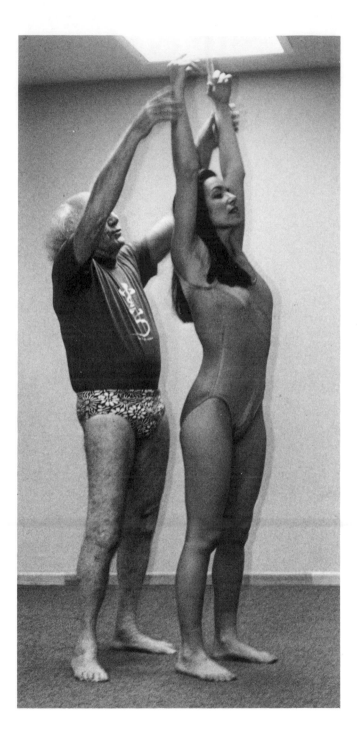

Standing in this free, elongated position
takes the pressure
off the lower back.
This new feeling of elongation
will soon be powerful enough so the
old holding patterns will be pushed
in the background when these
new positive patterns take over.

After sitting and standing several times,
the height of inhalation will feel as though
your head is going up towards the ceiling.
Standing and walking will then become
    effortless activities.

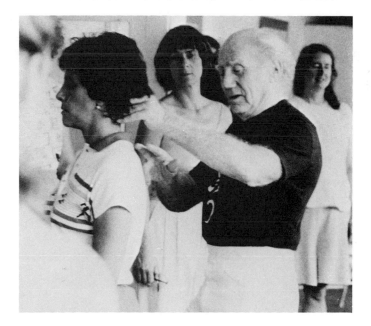

Repeat the postural movements,
and resume walking around the room several times.
Continue this sequence so you can be in
proper postural position as you walk.
The movements with the chair
and the walking are equally important,
especially in the acute stage
of a lower back problem.
Do not push your limits in order to
determine if you still have pain—
this recalls pain, and can cause muscle spasm.

The principle of moving in rhythm can also
facilitate other activities such as
        getting in and out of a car
        or getting dressed.
The pleasure from feeling at ease in standing in your
        personal, perfect posture
        can benefit all phases of your life.

Shifting Weight

Whenever you are on your feet,
you are constantly losing and recovering balance.
Even when you think you are standing "still,"
fine balance is employed.
The act of recovering your balance to prevent a fall
is a reflex response.
It occurs unconsciously.
Developing and improving balance
can increase your sense of
body awareness and coordination.

The soles of our feet contain a large number of
touch receptors which respond to pressure.
Shifting the weight on the feet is one way to
stimulate these receptors,
    which heightens body awareness and balance.

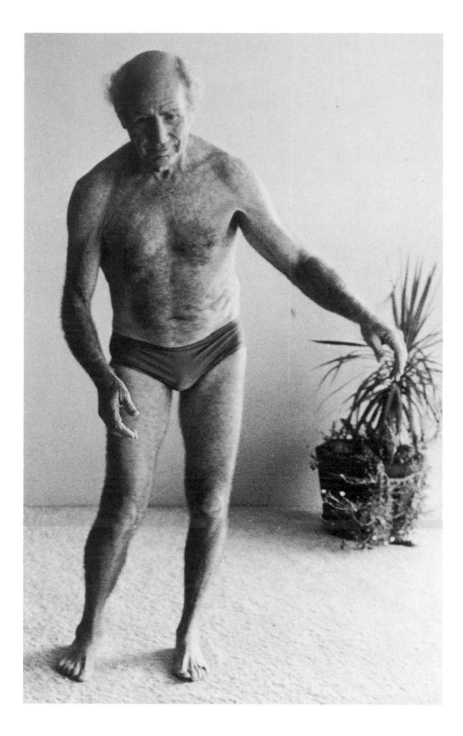

Stand with your feet about shoulder width apart
with the knees slightly bent.
Shift your weight moving from side to side
so that you feel the pressure change
from the inside to the outside of your feet.
Both feet always remain in contact with the floor.
The hips do not swing.
   Simply feel the bottom of your feet.

Shift your weight to each side
only to the point where
   you are not fighting balance.
If you feel yourself tightening,
or lifting one foot off the floor,
then decrease the amount of movement.
Be intimate with the feeling in the bottom of your feet.
Feel the difference in pressure as you
stimulate all of the tactile receptors in your feet.

You can also shift your weight forward and back.
When you lean forward,
feel your toes dig into the floor or carpet.
When you lean back,
feel your buttock and back muscles tighten a bit.
Never shift past the point where you must fight balance.

I always use this approach of
shifting weight to teach balance
to my paralyzed patients.
In order to walk,
    one must develop the
    use of their reflexes so that
    balance becomes an automatic pattern.

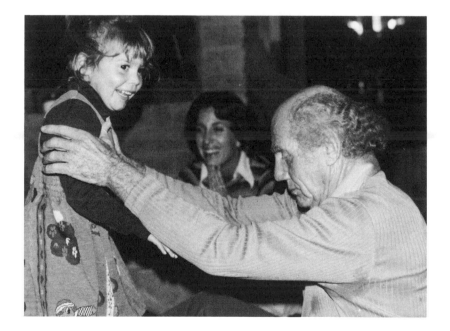

Use the shifting of weight to
keep your entire body free and fluid.
This subtle feeling of pressure in your feet
can bring you into
        hook-up.
It can be done anywhere,
and is especially useful if you are
        waiting in line at the store or bank.

The subtle shifting of weight on your feet
will bring you into
a state of nothingness.
And this state of nothingness
        is everything.

Side Stretch

A continuation of the shifting of weight
is the side stretch.
Clasp your hands over your head and
stretch up high.
The arms are straight, yet relaxed, and
keep them close to your ears.
    There is no effort.

Shift all of your weight onto your left foot,
so that you could lift your right foot
off of the floor.
Let the hip swing out to the left as the
arms stretch to the right.
This will elongate the left side of your body.

Shift all of your weight onto the right foot and
allow your hip to swing out to the right
as the arms stretch to the left,
elongating the right side of your body.

Make the movement long and lovely.

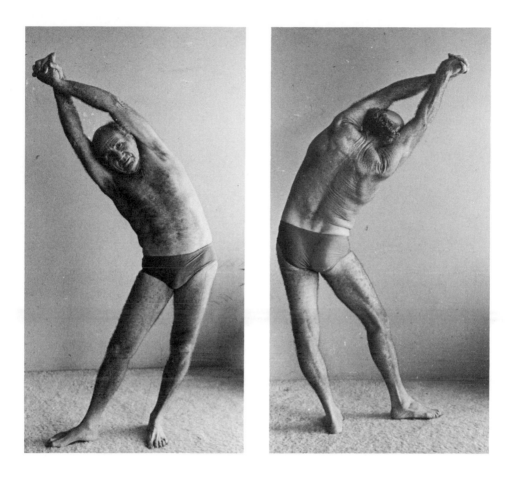

The side stretch is a long, beautiful excursion
from your hands to your heels.
Feel and be part of this length and beauty

Continue shifting your weight and
moving from side to side in rhythm.
    If this movement is done rhythmically,
    it isn't tiring.
    This stretch is done slowly and
    in hook-up.
Allow the rhythm to develop as
you continue to shift your weight.

There is no pain. There is no discomfort.
Just a pleasant sensation of
shifting the hips and the
weight on your feet in rhythm.
Ask the questions,
   "What is softer? What is freer?
   What is longer?" and
you will find yourself going into hook-up,
thus developing an effortless quality in the movement.

Allow this rhythmic stretch to
pleasure your body/mind with the feeling of
length and loveliness.

Arm Mentastics

Tensions, pains and discomforts arising in the
neck, shoulders, upper back and arms
can be alleviated by doing arm Mentastics.
The feeling and benefits of arm Mentastics come from
feeling and playing with the
weight of the arm and hand.

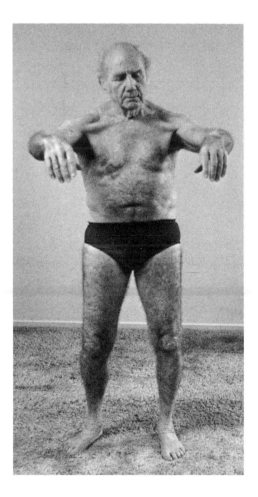

Slowly raise your arms up in front of you
with the elbows and wrists
relaxed and slightly bent.
Bring them up to chest height
    with the palms down.
    Feel the weight of your arms.

Then allow the weight and heaviness
of your arms to drop and swing down
by your sides.

Again, slowly raise your arms in front of you.
Be part of the weight.
Feel your arms so heavy that
you can hardly keep them up.
Being intimate with this feeling of weight
    can bring you into
    hook-up.

Allow the arms to swing down by your sides.
Do not drive them down.
Gravity will take care of the arms
    falling and swinging.
You, consciously,
    have nothing to do with the movement.

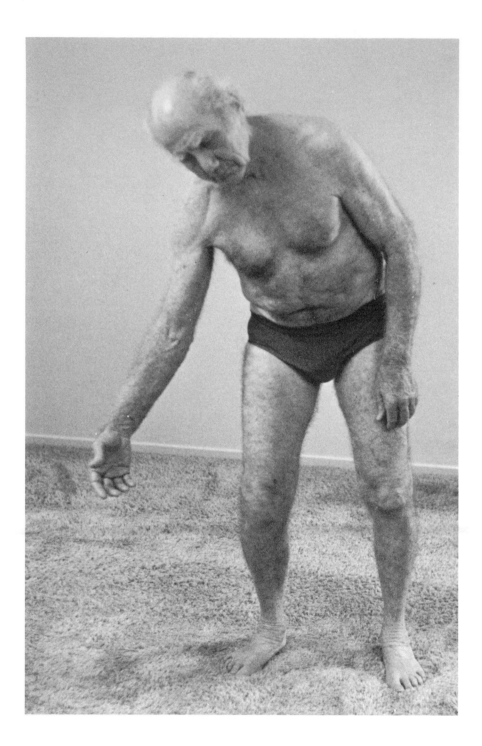

Choose the arm that feels the freest and
allow the weight of the arm to
    hang down from the shoulder
    close to your leg.
Gravity and the heaviness from the sheer
weight of the arm will
    allow it to hang.
This alone creates a subtle stretching and
opening in the neck and shoulders.
Then, bend the elbow and drop the arm once.
Pause a moment…; then ask,
    "Well…how did it feel?"
Be part of the feeling. Continue asking,
    "What is freer than that?"
  This process will bring you into a
    fine state of hook-up.

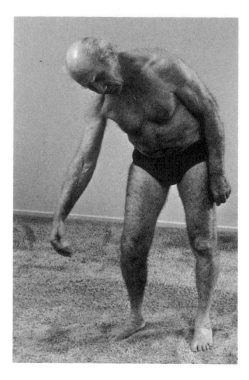

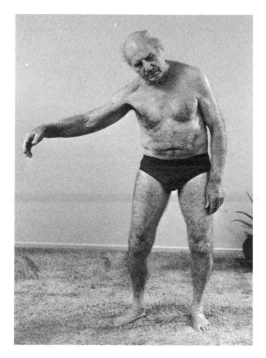

150

It is not your words that will develop the feeling.
You will develop by
EXPERIENCING the feeling.
Expect an answer.
The answer may sound something like,
    "Oh, yes, this feels lighter.
    This is easier and better."

Create a shimmering in the arms by
feeling and playing with the
    weight of the thumb.
You can develop a finer feeling of the
weight of the thumb by
positioning and moving your hand as if you are
    strumming a guitar.
All of the fingers become part of the movement.

You will feel that the shimmering activates the
muscles of the forearm as well as the
elbow and muscles in the upper arm.
The shimmering goes from the thumb to the shoulder.
Do not try to make the arm muscles bounce.
Allow the shimmering to occur as if
you are softly saying,
    "Hi, muscles."

My students often ask me,
    "Where is the movement coming from?
    Is it coming from my shoulder,
    my arm, or my hand?"
I say to them,
    "It is coming from your mind.
    And if the movement does not
    originate from your mind,
    then you are trying too hard.
    It is a happening."

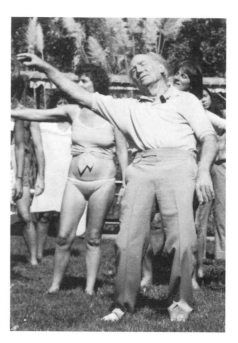

Allow the momentum to swing the arm
up and down in front.
Feel the space you can create in the
shoulder and chest as you
    shimmer your arm out to the side.
As you bring the arm up,
the elbow bends at the height of the movement
    from the weight of the arm.

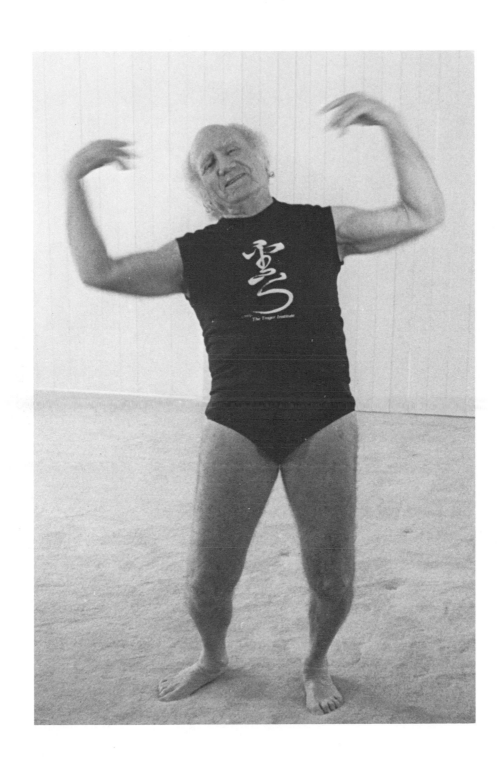

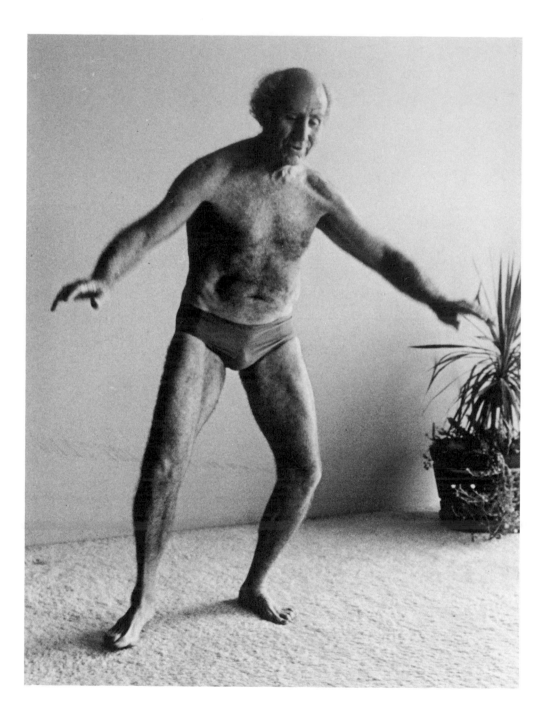

If you feel tension coming into
any part of your arm or hand,
    then slow down the movement.
You cannot feel the subtle shimmerings when
    moving too fast.
Allow the movement to be a
soft, steady, rhythmic, quieting motion
    as if you were putting a baby to sleep.

Repeat the arm Mentastics to the other side.
There will be an automatic transference of the
feeling of lightness
to the other arm.
You might even ask and recall,
    "How did it feel to do it
    on the other side?"

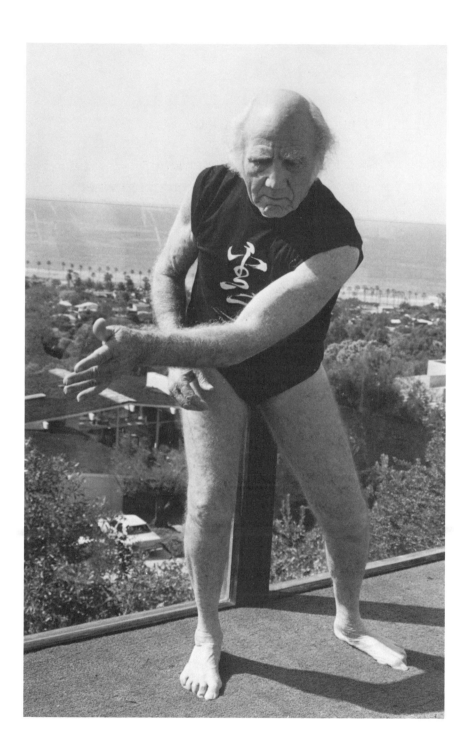

To develop a deeper and finer sense of
lightness and hook-up,
bring your arm across your body as if you are
    pushing the air away.
There are no hesitations.
Sustain this feeling in the arm.
There is no strength.
    How lightly can you push the air away…

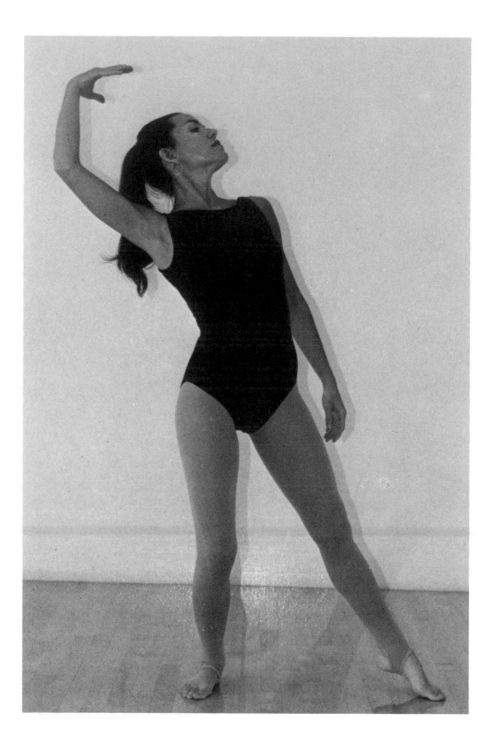

Combine this movement with a swing of your arm
up and around the head
as if you are brushing your hair.
   It is a continuous movement.
This movement can bring a sense of
beauty and softness into your
      arms and chest.

Enjoy the lightness and
agelessness in your arms.
The lighter the tissue,
the more ageless it becomes.
Discover and play with your potential for
moving in a better way.

   Play.
      Feel.
         Be there.

Arm Swings

A sense of freedom in the entire body,
especially in the chest and upper back,
can be felt by doing the arm swings.
The complete, effortless swinging of the arms
can bring you into a oneness with
the weight of your arms.
    This feeling of oneness
    can bring you into hook-up.

Stand with your feet about shoulder width apart
with the knees slightly bent.
The arms are hanging down by your sides
as you begin to gently swing
so that the arms wrap around your body.
Feel the momentum from the weight of your arms
    doing the movement.

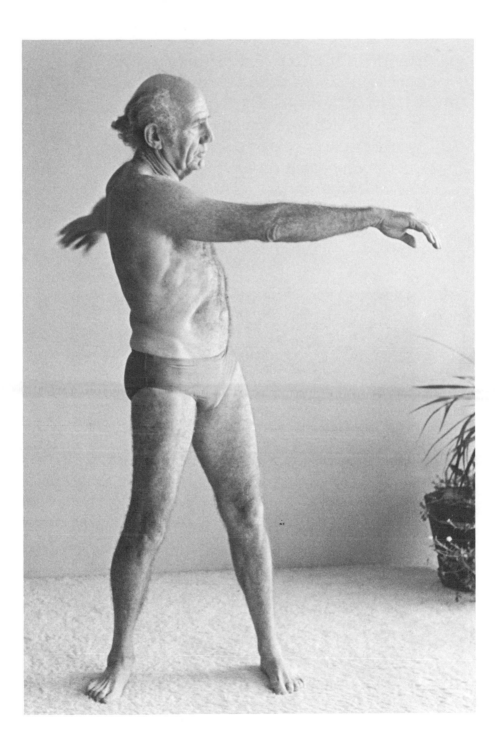

As you swing, let your eyes follow the back hand.
Keep your feet in contact with the floor.
Continue to swing as you raise your arms with
the palms facing down.
   Feel your little fingers cut through the air.
The level of the arms is below shoulder height,
as though your hands can wrap around your body and
come under the armpit
If any tension or discomfort develops,
   then lower the arms.

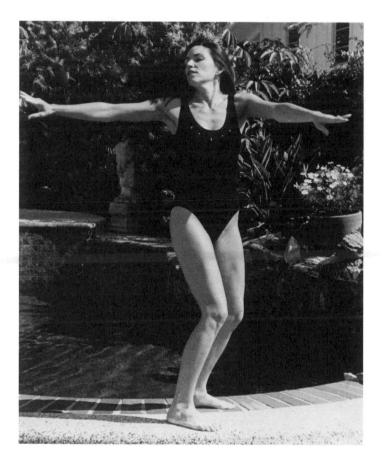

Do not place your arms in position.
    Allow them to swing.
It is a broad, sweeping movement.
    It is a feeling of abandonment.

Do the movement slow enough to
feel the weight of the arms take you.
As your eyes follow the back hand,
make sure that it does not drop down.

Both arms stay level during the swing.

Feel the opening in the chest and upper back.
Sense the rotation and freedom in the spine.
Be aware of the effects of the arm swings from your
feet up to your head.
This lovely gesture is moving you towards agelessness.

The Windmill

The windmill is a movement that
utilizes the momentum of the weight of the arms
in a similar manner as the arm swings.
It is fantastic for freeing the waist, ribs, and hips.

Bend over from the waist and just hang.
Keep the knees slightly bent.
Let go of the head so it is also hanging.
Throw your arms back to swing.
Follow your back hand with your eyes,
which allows more of a twist to happen.

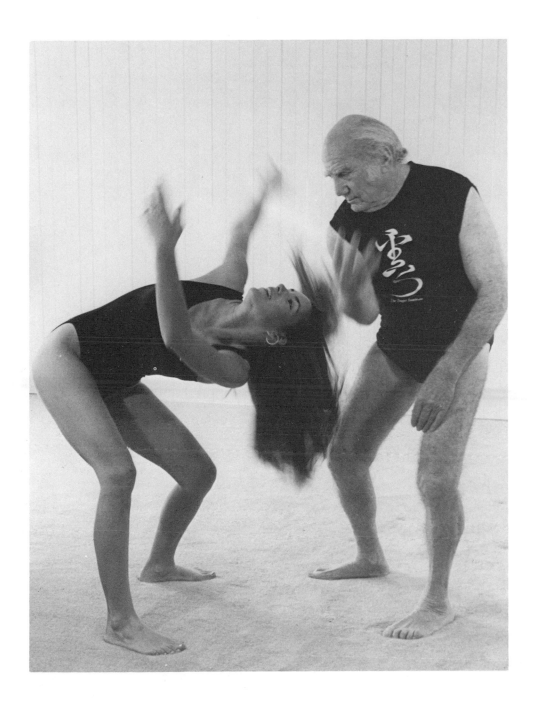

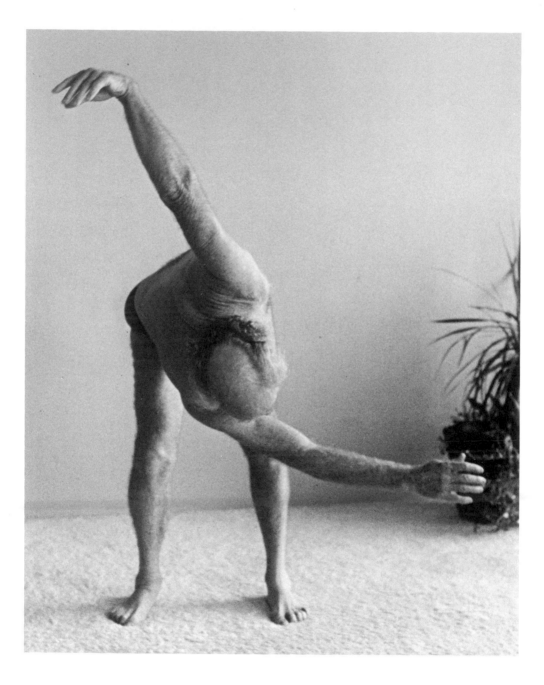

The trunk does not swing or dip up and down.
Keep your trunk centered as
you rotate around.
If you feel dizzy,
slow down in doing the movement.
Come up and out of the windmill slowly
so as not to encourage
dizziness or to lose your balance.

The windmill is done in rhythm as
the arms swing back and up towards the ceiling.
Enjoy the process of
discovering the freedom in your body/mind.

Expand The Chest & Develop Hook-Up

Place your fingertips at the pubic bone
keeping the knees soft. (see #1)
Slide your fingers up the abdomen
giving the tissue of the belly an
    uplifting feeling.

Continue to slide up and under the ribs.
As you slide up,
pull in your abdominal wall as though it could
touch the front of your spine. (see #2)
The feeling for this movement comes from
the abdomen and chest.

Let your chest be your inspiration for expression.

Take this feeling of openness and beauty
past your abdomen and chest
by bringing your arms up and around.
Keep your knees soft. (see #3)

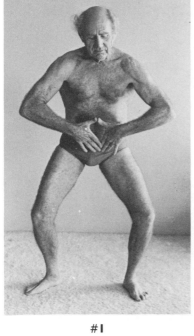

#1

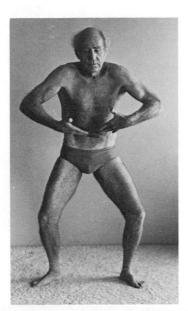

#2

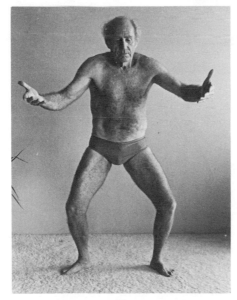

#3

169

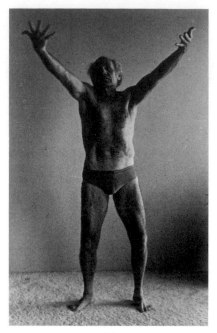

#4

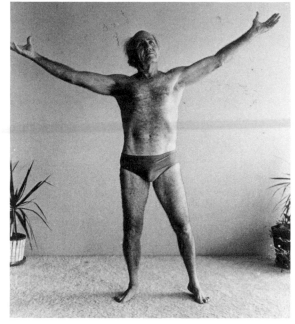

#5

170

The arms wind up in front in an open position
with the palms up. (#4 & #5)
The meaning to this movement could be,
    "I have so much within myself.
    Here . . . you take some.
    I can afford to freely give
    this wonderful feeling away."
Enjoy the feeling of the palms facing up
with the sensation of giving.

As you continue this movement,
feel all of the air coming in.
It is a very expansive and deep sense of being.
Allow the rhythm and sense of freely giving out,
deepen your experience and
    expression of hook-up.

Subtle Form of Breathing

Sit comfortably in a chair or lie down on a bed.
Feel how effortlessly you can take air in as you breathe.
  It is so simple…so nothing.
Let the air come in. Do not try to take a deep breath.

This subtle form of breathing can bring one
into a deep state of hook-up.
  There is zero effort. Do not try to do it right.
  Be part of the air coming in
  to the depth that can happen.
Exhalation will occur automatically.

Feel the relaxation envelope your entire body
as you softly breathe in;
inhaling with conscious simplicity.

It all comes down to nothing;
without doing anything about it at all.
There are all degrees of depth of
Mentastics and hook-up.

This is my ultimate experience in Mentastics.
I have no idea of
where it will develop from here…
    What is better than this…?

Photographic Credits

The Publisher gratefully acknowledges permission to use the photographs in this book, for which all rights are reserved to the photographers. Listing is alphabetical by photographer, followed by the page numbers in the book (designating page order, from left to right and top to bottom, as a, b, c, following the number).

Nina Amory: 94 (c, d, & e)

Judith Beatie: 45

Ralph Chaney: 43, 99 (a & b), 108, 146, 148, 150 (a & b)

Carla Chotzen: 62

Helene Closset: 18, 44, 82, 98, 103, 135

Daniel L. Fishman: 78, 120, 130, 132 (a & b), 153, 156, 162, 165

Tom Frankenberg: 35, 134

Cathy Guadagno: 49, 58, 66, 68, 92, 127

Robert Hammond: 86, 94 (a & b), 158

Rollin Inman: 61, 96

Joan Phillips: 24, 30, 33, 38, 41, 42, 46, 48, 50, 55, 57, 84, 88, 90, 106, 110, 112, 116, 118 (a & b), 122, 124, 126, 138, 143 (a & b), 154, 161, 166, 169 (a, b, c), 170

Emily Trager: 104

University of California at Los Angeles Laboratory: 70, 72, 74, 76 (a & b)

For further information regarding Mentastics ℠, please contact:
The Trager Institute
10 Old Mill Road
Mill Valley, California 94941

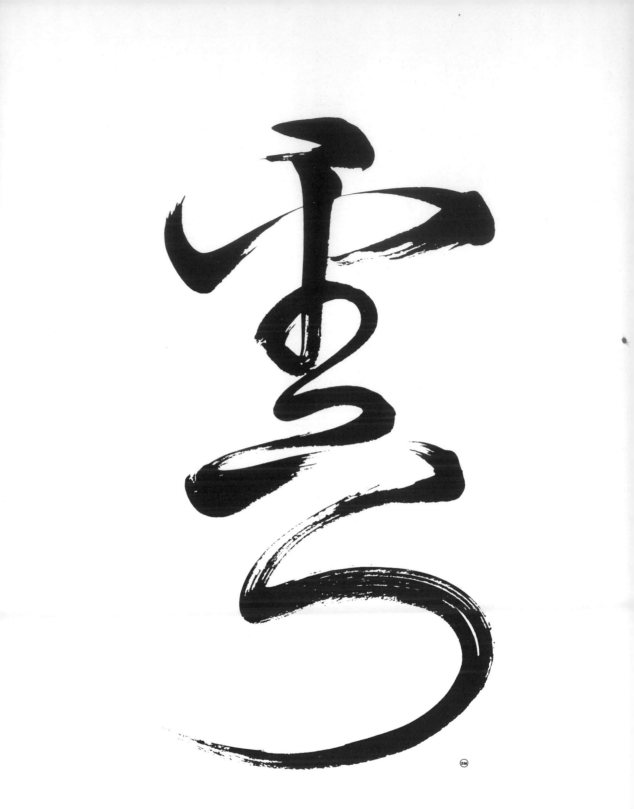

Dancing Cloud, calligraphy by Al Chung-liang Huang, created for The Trager Institute for Psychophysical Integration and Mentastics